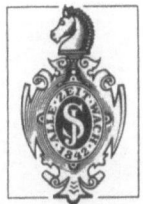

G. Bönner   K.H. Rahn

Prostacyclin and Hypertension

With 49 Figures and 4 Tables

Springer-Verlag Berlin Heidelberg New York
London Paris Tokyo Hong Kong

Priv.-Doz. Dr. Gerd Bönner
Medizinische Universitätsklinik II
Städtische Krankenanstalten Merheim
Ostmerheimer Straße 200
D-5000 Köln 91, FRG

Professor Dr. Karl-Heinz Rahn
Medizinische Poliklinik der Universität Münster
Albert-Schweitzer-Straße 33
D-4400 Münster, FRG

Translation from the second revised edition in German

ISBN-13: 978-3-540-52140-2   e-ISBN-13: 978-3-642-95608-9
DOI: 10.1007/ 978-3-642-95608-9

The use of general descriptive names, registered names, trademarks, etc. in this publi-
cations does not imply, even in the absence of a specific statement, that such names are
exempt from the relevant protective laws and regulations and therefore free for general
use.

Product Liability: The publisher can give no guarantee for information about drug dosage
and application thereof contained in this book. In every individual case the respective
user must check its accuracy by consulting other pharmaceutical literature.

Preface to the Second Edition

The aim of present-day treatment of hypertension is no longer regarded merely as the effective reduction of blood pressure, but as the ever-increasing application of new therapeutic principles to prevent such consequences of hypertension as left heart hypertrophy, medial hypertrophy of the vessels and arteriosclerosis. In this context special attention has been directed to stimulation of the endogenous vasocilator hormonal systems such as the prostaglandins. The great interest in our book, which has meanwhile appeared in a French edition, seems to confirm this trend and has encouraged us to include in the book the new findings published in the last twelve months. These changes and additions maintain the current status of the book and provide an even more complete survey of the available information about prostacyclin in hypertension. We wish to thank all those colleagues who have made useful suggestions for this second edition, as well as Springer-Verlag and its associates, who ensured a uniformly smooth passage in the production of the book.

Cologne and Münster, January 1990   Gerd Bönner
Karl-Heinz Rahn

Preface to the First Edition

Diseases of the heart and circulation currently constitute the commonest causes of death in our population. Hypertension, as evidenced by a pathologic increase in blood pressure, is one of the most important risk factors. Primary hypertension can be established in about 15% of adults. Patients with hypertension usually feel well subjectively and only rarely complain of symptoms. It therefore often happens that hypertension is discovered only after the manifestation of complications such as myocardial infarction, cerebrovascular accident and renal failure. There are now available for the treatment of primary hypertension numerous groups of drugs which, however, usually reduce blood pressure only nonspecifically. At the present time a causal therapy is still not possible, for despite intensive research, the pathogenesis of primary (idiopathic) hypertension still remains altogether obscure. In recent years, diverse variations in the activities of the vasoactive hormones have been proposed as the cause of the increased blood pressure. Yet, although the significance of the renin-angiotensin system for the development of renovascular hypertension has been clearly demonstrated, it has remained difficult to evaluate the role of the various vasoconstrictor and vasodilator prostaglandins in the pathogenesis of primary hypertension. Amongst the prostaglandins, prostacyclin (PGI_2) appears to be particularly important for blood pressure regulation since it is regarded as a specific vascular prostaglandin formed preferentially in the endothelia and smooth muscle cells of the vessels and as one of the most potent local vasodilators.

It is the aim of this book to demonstrate the special relationship of the "vascular prostaglandin", i.e. prostacyclin, to circulatory regulation, with special reference to the lesions investigated hitherto in hypertension. The authors are well aware that in a review of this kind, even with due attention to all the accessible references, no conclusive judgment can be reached as to the significance of prostacyclin in the pathogenesis of hypertension. However, this synopsis will certainly help every interested physician and research worker to from his own view of the physiologic and pathophysiologic significance of the vascular prostaglandin PGI_2.

We would like to take this opportunity of thanking all those who have contributed so energetically to the completion of this book.

Cologne and Münster, July 1988   Gerd Bönner
                                        Karl-Heinz Rahn

Contents

List of Abbreviations

A	=	angiotensin
A'gen	=	angiotensinogen
AA	=	arachidonic acid
ACE	=	angiotensin I converting enzyme
ADH	=	antidiuretic hormone
ATP	=	adenosine triphosphate
BK	=	bradykinin
cAMP	=	cyclic adenosine-3',5'-monophosphate
Cap	=	captopril
CE	=	cholesterol ester
CHOL	=	cholesterol
FFA	=	free fatty acids
SCP	=	sterol carrier protein
DOCA	=	deoxycorticosterone acetate
HCO	=	hydrogenated coconut oil
HDL	=	high density lipoprotein
HPETE	=	hydroxy-peroxy-eicosatetraenic acid
HPLC	=	high-performance liquid chromatography
HR	=	heart rate
Indo	=	indomethacin
Kal	=	kallikrein
LDL	=	low density lipoprotein
LT	=	leukotriene
NE	=	norepinephrine
NR	=	normotensive rats
P_D	=	diastolic arterial blood pressure
PDGF	=	platelet-derived growth factor
PG	=	prostaglandin
P_s	=	systolic arterial blood pressure
R	=	Dahl salt-resistant rats
RR	=	blood pressure
SHR	=	spontaneously hypertensive rats
S	=	Dahl salt-sensitive rats

TX = thromboxane
WKY = Wistar-Kyoto rats

1 Introduction

The regulation of systemic blood pressure is based on multiple central and peripheral regulatory mechanisms, among which the vasoactive hormonal systems play a not insignificant part. In the past it was particularly the hormonal systems with an active vasopressor effect such as the renin-angiotensin system, the mineralocorticoids, catecholamines and the antidiuretic hormone that attracted the greatest attention in hypertension research. For a long period an excessive importance was attached to the vasopressor hormones as the essential cause of arterial hypertension, but the importance of vasodepressor hormone systems such as the kallikrein-kinin system and the prostaglandins remained unappreciated for many years, and a deficiency of vasodepressor agents was seldom considered as a pathogenetic factor in the development of hypertension. This is the more surprising since the blood pressure-lowering action of the kallikrein-kinin system (the "F substance") had been discovered by FREY and KRAUT [74] as far back as 1926.

Just a few years later, in 1930, the first studies of KURZROCK and LIEB [135] were published which showed that human seminal fluid can exert a relaxing effect on the human uterine muscle. In 1933, GOLDBLATT [87] discovered the lipidlike nature of this substance and demonstrated its blood pressure-lowering effect. A year later the studies of VON EULER confirmed the blood pressure-reducing action of the seminal fluid, and in 1935 he gave this substance the name "prostaglandin" because of its supposed origin in the prostate [62]. Finally, in 1962, BERGSTRÖM'S team succeeded in elucidating the structure of the first prostaglandins, PGE as well as PGF$_1$ and PGF$_2$ [18]. The following years saw the rapid discovery of further prostaglandins as products of cyclooxygenase which, in accordance with a suggestion of COREY et al. [42], have been grouped as eicosanoids (molecules with 20 carbon atoms, Fig. 1). Prostacyclin is one of the most recently discovered eicosanoids and has a very short history. The first evidence of the prostacyclin discovered later was found by TS'AO in 1970 [262] in studies in which he observed that complete segments of blood vessels did not induce platelet aggregation, whereas collagen isolated from the same vessels did produce immediate aggregation. In 1976 the team of VANE [94] succeeded in identifying the aggregation-inhibiting substance of the vessels as a prostaglandin. Initially, they called this prosta-

1

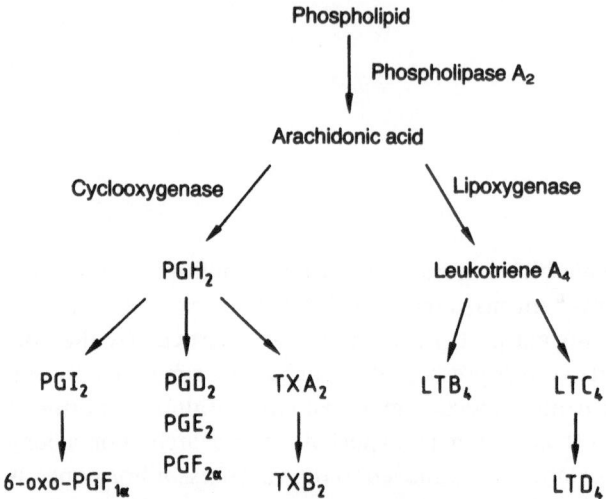

Fig. 1. Cyclooxygenase- and lipoxygenase-controlled arachidonic acid metabolism (*PG*, prostaglandin; *TX*, thromboxane; *LT*, leukotriene)

glandin PGX, but later this was adapted to the conventional nomenclature and the name defined as prostaglandin I_2 (PGI$_2$) [126]. The appellation "PGI" is based on the sequence of discovery (structural elucidation after that of PGH) and the index "2" on the number of double bonds in the side chains. The term "prostacyclin" was chosen on the basis of the double ring structure. In 1982 VANE was awarded the Nobel Prize for the discovery of prostacyclin.

2 Biochemistry and Pharmacology of Prostacyclin

2.1 Biochemical Specification and Metabolism

Structure
The structural elucidation of prostacyclin (PGI_2) showed that this substance is to be regarded as a typical cyclooxygenase product of the eicosanoids. The chemical structure of prostacyclin (Fig. 2) is described as 9-deoxo-6,9α-epoxy-delta^5-$PGF_{1\alpha}$ [289].

Biosynthesis
The biosynthesis of prostacyclin originates from arachidonic acid. Cyclooxygenase and peroxidase, with the aid of oxygen, convert the arachidonic acid via 11-HPETE and PGG_2 into PGH_2, which serves as the substrate for prostacyclin synthetase [175]. The latter is identical with membrane-fixed prostaglandin-endoperoxide-6,9-oxycyclase and is very probably a hemoprotein with a molecular weight of 52 000 daltons [48]. It catalyzes the formation of the double ring structure of prostacyclin from PGH_2 [235]. Prostacyclin synthetase exhibits a broad pH optimum and is stimulated by a soluble cell substance not so far characterized in detail [298].

Metabolism
Prostacyclin itself is a poorly stable substance and rapidly inactivated. In vivo, at a pH of 7.4 and at 37 °C, its average biochemical half-life is only 3 min [56]. However, in vitro the half-life as measured by platelet aggregation is significantly higher, in the region of several hours [210]. The breakdown of prostacyclin takes place mainly in the circulation, liver and kidney, but not in the lungs, so that there is no noteworthy pulmonary clearance, and significant arteriovenous differences are not demonstrable [289]. The main breakdown of prostacyclin is not based on any specific enzymatic stage, as there is initially formed the essentially stable hydrolyis product 6-oxo-$PGF_{1\alpha}$. This is further converted by β-oxidation into the end-product 2,3-dinor-6-oxo-$PGF_{1\alpha}$ which, like 6-oxo-$PGF_{1\alpha}$, is eliminated by the kidneys (Fig. 3).

However, inactivation of prostacyclin can also be effected enzymatically by 15-hydroxy-prostaglandin-dehydrogenase. The 15-oxo-PGI_2 so formed is

3

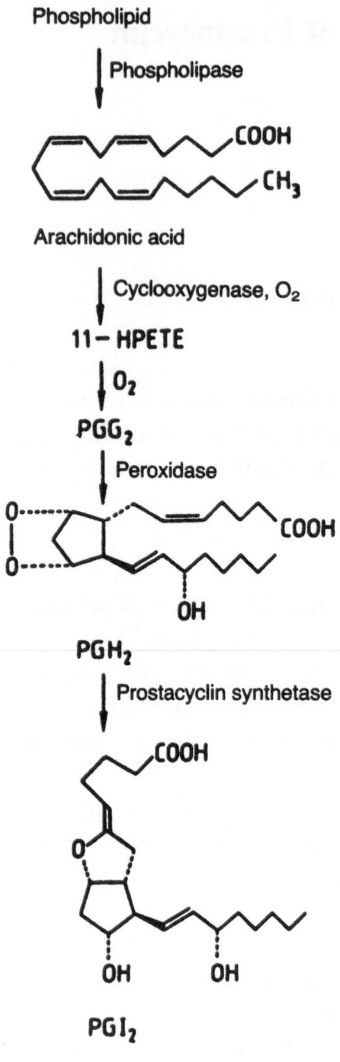

Phospholipid

↓ Phospholipase

COOH
CH₃

Arachidonic acid

↓ Cyclooxygenase, O₂

11 – HPETE

↓ O₂

PGG₂

↓ Peroxidase

COOH
OH

PGH₂

↓ Prostacyclin synthetase

COOH
OH   OH

PGI₂

Fig. 2. Prostacyclin synthesis from phospholipids

immediately converted by hydrolysis in a second stage to 6,15-dioxo-PGF$_{1\alpha}$, which is transformed by delta^{13}-reductase into 13,14-dihydro-6,15-dioxo-PGF$_{1\alpha}$. After a rapid β-oxidation to 13,14-dihydro-2,3-dinor-6,15-dioxo-PGF$_{1\alpha}$ this endproduct is then likewise eliminated by the kidneys. However, besides this breakdown into biologically inactive products, prostacyclin can also be converted into another and still very biologically potent prostaglandin (Fig. 4). In the liver, kidneys and platelets there is present 9-hydroxy-prosta-glandin-dehydrogenase which converts prostacyclin into stable 6-keto-PGE₁

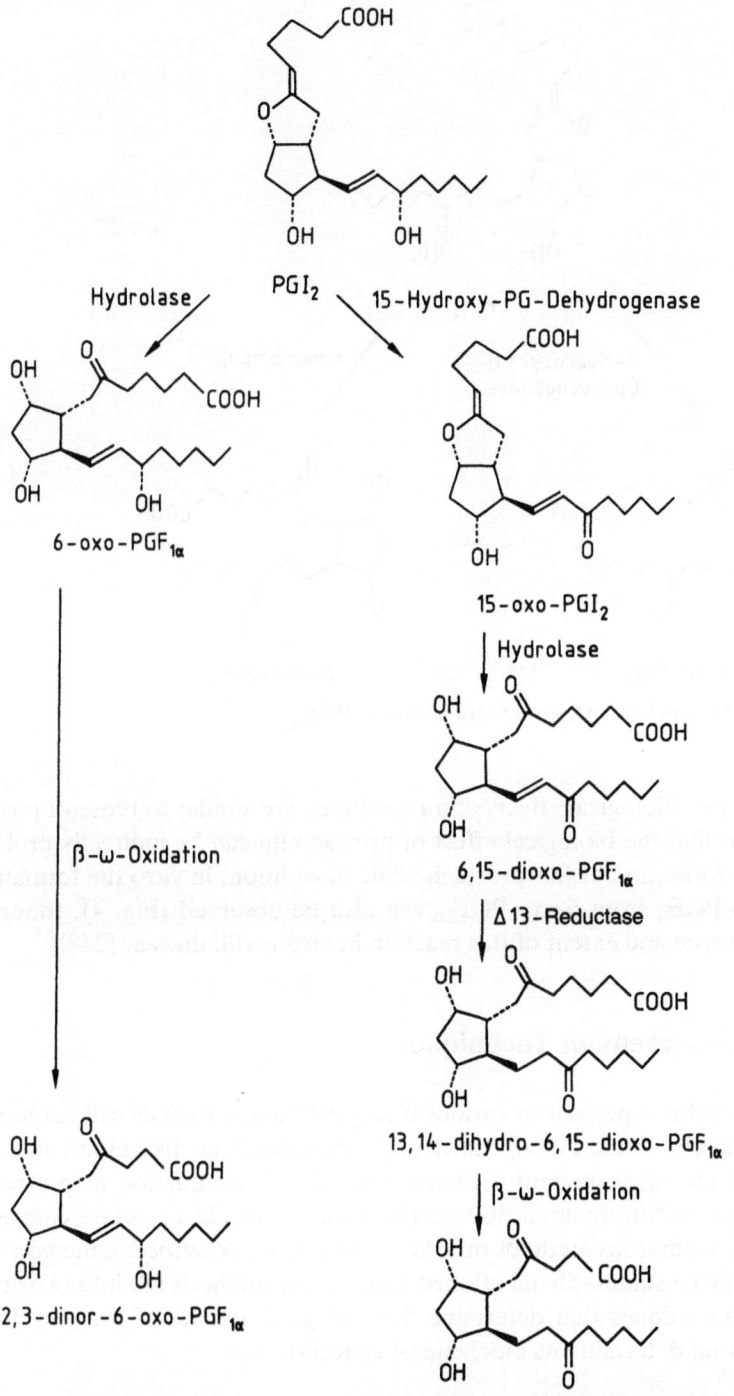

Fig. 3. Metabolism of prostacyclin to inactive breakdown products

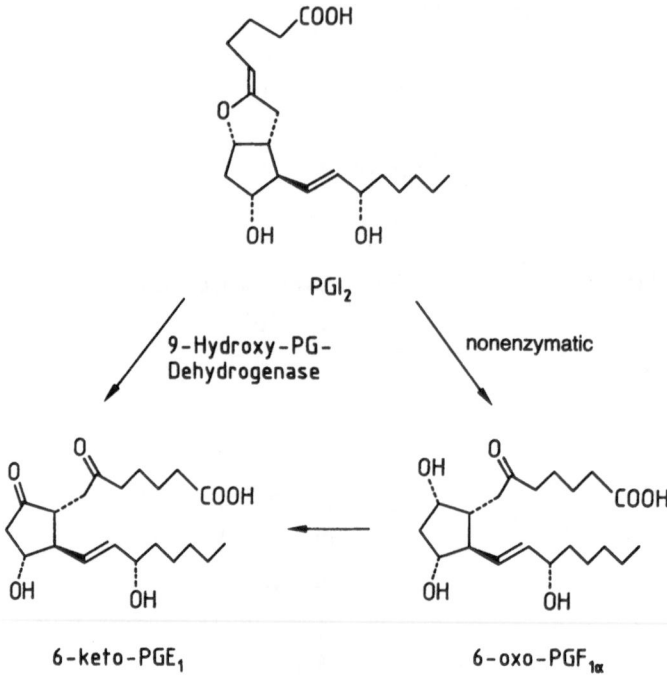

Fig. 4. Metabolism of prostacyclin to 6-keto-PGE$_1$

[299]. The biological effects of 6-keto-PGE$_1$ are similar to those of prostacyclin, so that the biological effect of prostacyclin can be indirectly prolonged by the formation of this prostaglandin. In addition, in vitro the formation of 6-keto-PGE$_1$ from 6-oxo-PGF$_{1\alpha}$ can also be observed (Fig. 4), though the importance and extent of this reaction in vivo is still unclear [248].

2.2 Measurement Techniques

Prostacyclin is present in various biological media, such as cell cultures and their media, tissue homogenates and biological fluids like blood and urine. Hence the measurement techniques for the determination of prostacyclin must be uniformly applicable to the different media to obtain comparable values. Numerous methods of measurement were described in the past which will only be summarily mentioned here. These methods fall into two groups: those techniques that determine the biological activity of prostacyclin and those that determine its biochemical concentration.

Bioassay

The biological assay of prostacyclin can be established from its organ-specific effects. These include essentially the inhibition of platelet aggregation, the inhibition of serotonin liberation from activated platelets and the relaxation of the vascular smooth muscle in bioassay [25, 134]. These methods of measurement are relatively nonspecific because of possible interference with activity by other substances. The employment of specific prostacyclin antibodies or inhibitory prostacyclin analogues notably adds to the specificity of the bioassay and also allows more reliable findings with these techniques [247]. For the determination of the biological activity of circulating prostacyclin, the concentration of cyclic adenosine monophosphate in the platelets of fresh blood samples was measured with and without prostacyclin antibodies [111]. However, all these biological methods of measurement only allow indirect determination of prostacyclin by means of its activity, not of its absolute concentration. To improve the standardization of bioassays, uniform criteria have been proposed to monitor specificity [289]. These criteria require, on the one hand, a rapid reversal of PGI_2-like activity by inactivation within 30 s at 100 °C and pH 7.4, in 30 min at 25 °C or by acidification of the medium to pH 3, and on the other hand a maintained PGI_2-like activity with an environmental pH of over 9. In addition, it must be possible to influence this activity with specific prostacyclin antibodies as well as with inhibitors of cyclooxygenase and also prostacyclin synthetase.

Biochemical Assays

Methods allowing measurement of the actual concentration of prostacyclin are more specific. These include thin layer chromatography, radioimmunoassay and gas chromatography/mass spectroscopy. Currently, the most reliable separation of the different prostaglandins is by the high-performance liquid chromatography (HPLC) technique, which should be included in individual measurement techniques. These techniques can be used quantitatively, but have the great disadvantage, because of the short half-life of prostacyclin, of not determining prostacyclin itself, but often only its breakdown products such as 6-oxo-$PGF_{1\alpha}$. For this reason these techniques cannot provide reliable information as to the biological activity of prostacyclin, so that the decision between activity measurement in bioassay and biochemical determination of concentration depends on the experimental or clinical problem posed.

In laboratory routines the ability to determine prostacyclin itself is limited because of its short persistence. However, the conditions are more favourable with plasma samples stored immediately below -25 °C at pH 10. In these special circumstances the stability of prostacyclin can even be prolonged for weeks [235].

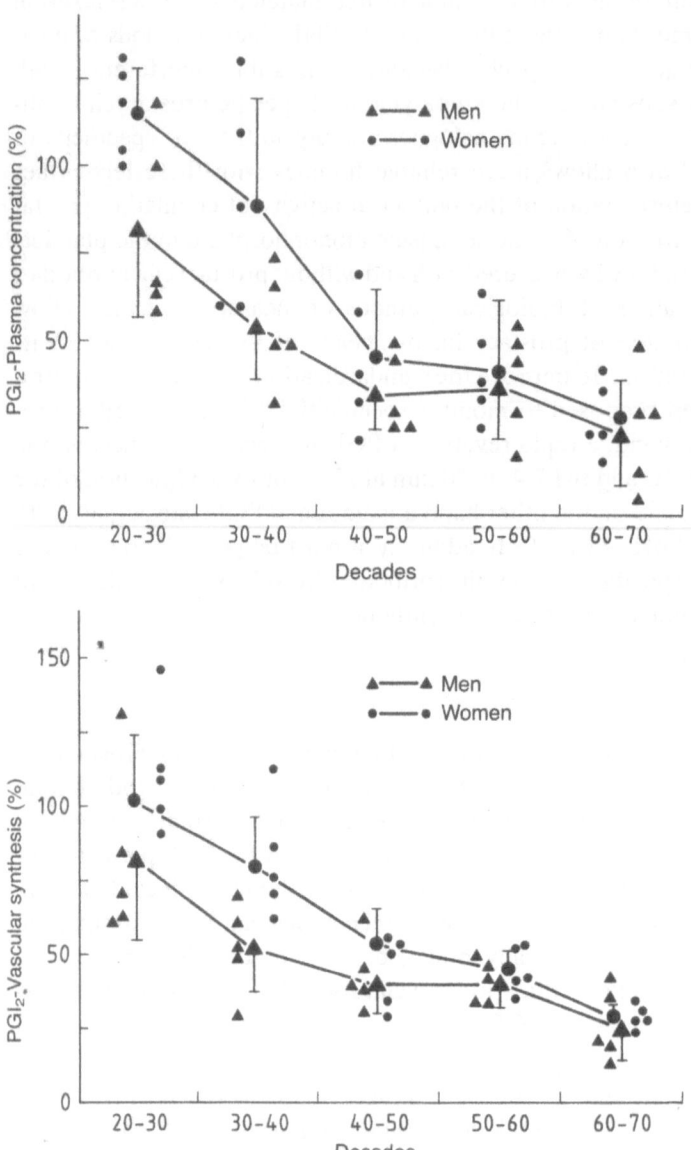

Fig. 5. Relation of vascular synthesis and plasma concentration of prostacyclin to age and sex (individual and mean values in five women and five men: 100 % corresponds to the value in the youngest group; $\bar{x} \pm$ SEM) [159]

Normal Values

The biosynthesis rate for prostacyclin of the entire organism is on average 60 pg/kg per min [234]. The normal plasma levels of prostacyclin are given in the literature as 5–18 ng/l, corresponding to 0.2–0.5 nmol/l [111, 220]. The concentrations of 6-oxo-PGF$_{1\alpha}$ vary around 300 ng/l [289]. The daily renal excretion of 6-oxo-PGF$_{1\alpha}$, the chief metabolite of prostacyclin, is specified as an average amount of 400 ng per day in healthy persons [92]. In women the plasma prostacyclin concentration is higher than in men. In both groups [159] prostacyclin synthesis in the tissues and the corresponding prostacyclin concentration in the blood decrease continuously with advancing age (Fig. 5).

2.3 Localization and Secretion

Localization of Prostacyclin Synthesis

The chief site of prostacyclin synthesis is the vessel wall, with special emphasis on its intimal portion. Though the intimal tissue represents only a small part (some 5%) of the vessel wall, it synthesizes over 40% of the prostacyclin [170] formed by the entire vessel wall (Fig. 6). The importance of the intima as a site of prostacyclin synthesis is even more important in view of the fact that some 32% of the PGH$_2$ is converted to prostacyclin in the intimal region, whereas the figure for the adventitia of the same vessels is less than 3% (Table 1). There is a wide variation in prostacyclin synthesis in the different vascular areas. For example, the human umbilical veins are capable

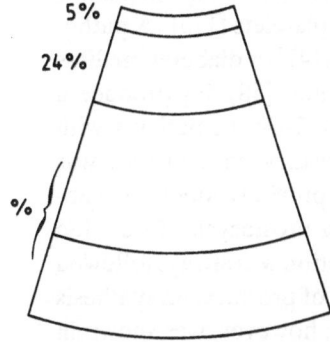

	Percentage	Absolute PGI$_2$-formation	Relative PGI$_2$-formation
Intima	5%	1,0 ng	20,0 ng/mg
Internal elastic lamina	24%	0,6 ng	2,5 ng/mg
Media and Adventitia	71%	1,1 ng	1,6 ng/mg
	100%	2,7 ng	2,7 ng/mg

Total prostacyclin produced by 1 mg of artery

Fig. 6. Absolute and relative prostacyclin formation per mg of tissue in the different layers of the vessel wall [170]

Table 1. Conversion of exogenous PGH_2 in prostacyclin in the different layers of an arterial wall ($\bar{x} \pm$ SEM) [100]

Layer of arterial wall	Percentage conversion of PGH_2 into PGI_2
Intimal cell suspension	$31,8 \pm 2,5\%$
Internal elastic lamina	$4,3 \pm 0,1\%$
Media	$3,9 \pm 0,9\%$
Adventitia	$2,7 \pm 0,9\%$

of forming prostacyclin rapidly in high concentrations, whereas the parallel umbilical arteries form scarcely any [108]. In the systemic circulation the conditions are reversed. Here the arteries, especially the aorta and large arteries, are capable of forming increased prostacyclin, whereas the veins exhibit only minor rates of prostacyclin synthesis [289]. In addition, prostacyclin synthesis has so far been demonstrated in the following extravascular tissues: the interstitial cells of the renal medulla [297], the glomeruli of the renal cortex [80], human adipocytes [219], the fibroblasts of the skin [9], the leukocytes [71] and the mucosal cells of the stomach [292]. Prostacyclin synthesis has also been demonstrated in the pituitary and the cerebral capillaries [86, 253]. Human platelets are not capable of forming prostacyclin, even if thromboxane metabolism is inhibited [188].

Vascular Prostacyclin Synthesis
The numerous sites of prostaglandin synthesis should not detract from the fact that the chief site of prostacyclin synthesis is the vascular endothelium. The vessel endothelia are capable of forming prostacyclin both from endogenous precursors and from the endoperoxides of platelets, which is indicative of an interesting interaction between vessel wall and platelets [175]. A pathological lesion of the endothelium, as in atherosclerosis [47] or diabetes mellitus [125], as well as artificial damage to the endothelium [58, 59] produce a marked decline in local prostacyclin synthesis (Figs. 7–9). In patients with diabetes mellitus [125] the decline in vascular prostacyclin synthesis was associated with a marked increase of a hitherto not precisely identified substance in the blood capable of definitely stimulating prostacyclin formation in healthy vessels (Fig. 8). Artificial de-endothelialization was always followed by a recurrent rise in the initially greatly reduced rate of prostacyclin synthesis by the damaged vessel wall. This recurrent increase, however, was shown in these pharmacological experiments to be independent of the state of the endothelium as it was observed to an equal extent in re-endothelialized vessels

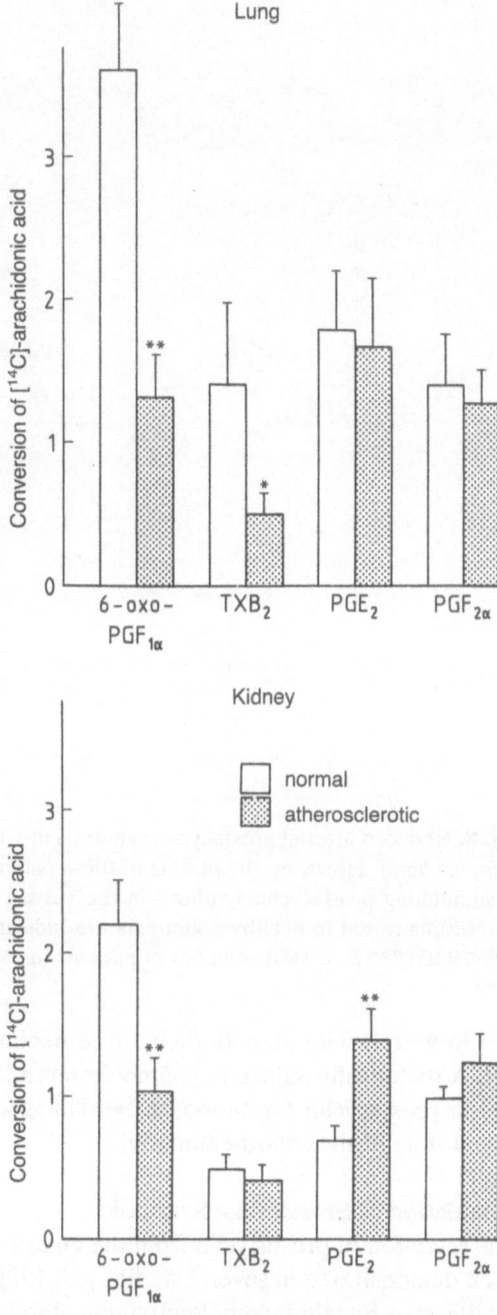

Fig. 7. Formation of 6-oxo-PGF$_{1\alpha}$, TXB$_2$, PGE$_2$ and PGF$_{2\alpha}$ in perfused normal and atherosclerotic lungs *(above)* and kidneys *(below)* in the rabbit. The total radioactivity transferred to the corresponding arachidonic acid metabolites is set out for each case. The total radioactivity obtained from the TLC plates was defined as 100% ($\bar{x} \pm$ SEM; * $P < 0.02$; ** $P < 0.005$) [47]

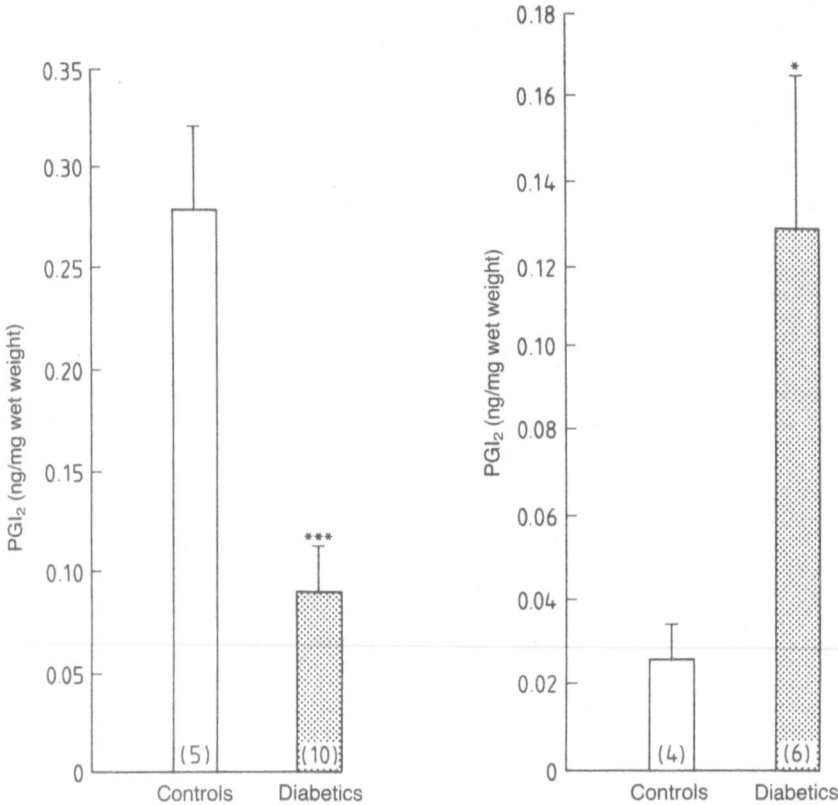

Fig. 8. Reduced arterial prostacyclin synthesis in vitro *(left panel)* in diabetic patients *(stippled bars)*. However, the plasma of these patients possesses an increased activity in stimulating prostacyclin synthesis in the vessels of healthy controls *(right panel)*. The results raised in healthy volunteers are indicated by the *open bars*. ($\bar{x}$ ± SEM; * $P < 0.05$; *** $P < 0.001$; number of patients in column) [125]

and in vessels with an endothelial-free neointima from smooth muscle [58, 59]. A dietetically induced hypercholesteremia (Fig. 9) prevented the return rise in prostacyclin formation in the damaged vessels independently of the actual state of the endothelium [59].

Stimulation of Prostacyclin Synthesis
The secretion of prostacyclin from the endothelial cells in the circulation has been demonstrated in several studies [69, 173], yet its regulation and clinical significance remain incompletely understood [33, 69, 220, 235]. Again, the multiple possibilities of stimulating prostacyclin synthesis (see below) do not permit agreement on a unitary stimulation mechanism. It is conceivable that

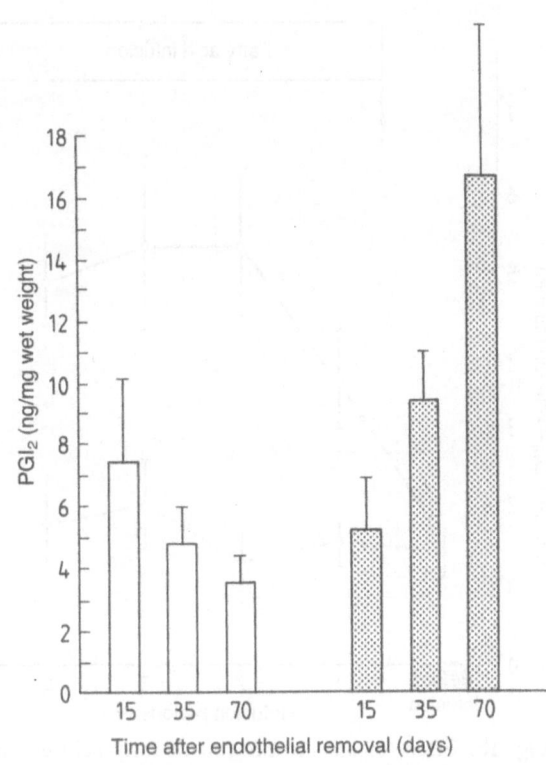

Fig. 9. Prostacyclin production in the re-endothelialized rabbit aorta 15, 35 and 70 days after balloon de-endothelialization. *Open bars* PGI_2 production in the aorta of rabbits receiving an egg-enriched diet; *stippled bars*, PGI_2 production in the aorta of rabbits receiving a normal diet ($\bar{x} \pm$ SEM) [59]

the increase in arachidonic acid metabolism may itself be decisive for the increase in prostacyclin synthesis. Whether prostacyclin is formed directly or another eicosanoid may depend to a certain extent on the specific prostaglandin metabolism of the actual cell type. Thus, in individual studies of vascular endothelia an increased rate of prostacyclin synthesis could be achieved merely by a general stimulation of prostaglandin synthesis. This was effected, on the one hand, by a stimulation of phospholipase A_2 by means of an increase in intracellular calcium, e.g. by the calcium ionophore A 23187, by direct calcium infusions or by inhibition of $Na^+ - K^+ -$ ATPase with ouabain [184, 186] and, on the other hand, by substitution of arachidonic acid in vitro [288] or fatty acid emulsion in vivo (Fig. 10) [60]. Yet stimulation of prostacyclin synthesis is produced not only by an increased supply of arachidonic acid and its precursors, but also by inhibition of thromboxane metabolism with specific inhibitors, such as CGS-13080, dazoxides or dazmegrel [11, 15]. It is very

13

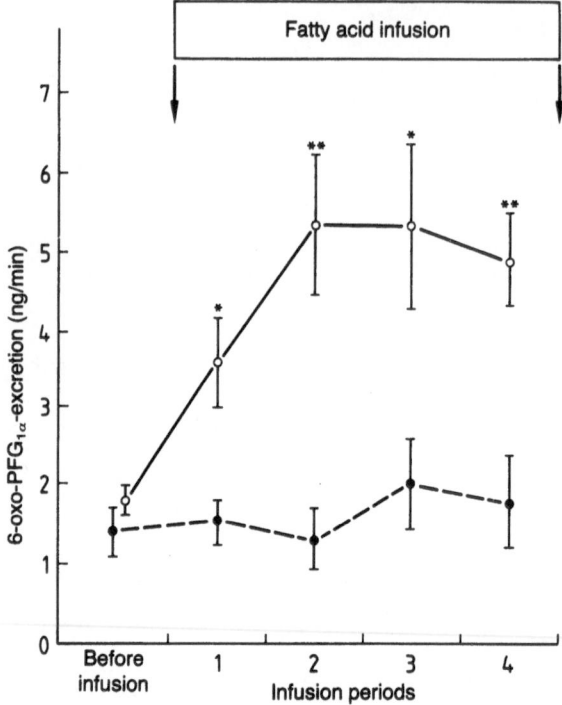

Fig. 10. Effect of an 8-h infusion of fatty acid emulsion on the renal excretion of immunoreactive 6-oxo-PGF$_{1\alpha}$ in five normal volunteers. Compared with placebo infusion, the fatty acid infusion stimulates renal 6-oxo-PGF$_{1\alpha}$ excretion. ($\bar{x} \pm$ SEM; o——o, fatty acid infusion; •– –•, placebo infusion; * $P < 0.06$; ** $P < 0.01$) [60]

probable that the inhibition of thromboxane synthetase causes an accumulation of the cyclic endoperoxides of cyclooxygenase metabolism, which leads to an increased supply of substrate for prostacyclin synthetase [155]. Moreover, prostacyclin formation may be stimulated by thrombin, collagen, trypsin or surface activation, as in operations [221, 234, 288]. An effective stimulator of endothelial prostacyclin synthetase is secreted from the platelets with the platelet-derived growth factor (PDGF). Even a concentration of 8 ng/ml of PDGF produces around a 74-fold increase in prostacyclin synthesis [43]. Among the vasoactive peptides, bradykinin and angiotensin II count as potent stimulators of prostacyclin formation [88, 120, 239] as do catecholamines [291] and the antidiuretic hormone (ADH) [234]. Histamine stimulates prostacyclin synthesis in endothelial cells via its H$_1$ receptors, but not in smooth muscle cells and fibroblasts [8, 10]. Norepinephrine stimulates prostacyclin formation only in the renal cells, not in the endothelia of the vessels [145,

14

289]. In human adipocytes prostacyclin synthesis can be increased by cAMP and isoproterenol [213]. Finally, it is a finding relevant to atherosclerosis research that HDL-cholesterol clearly increases prostacyclin formation in cultured cells, and is therefore capable of normalizing the suppression of cellular synthesis of prostacyclin produced by LDL-cholesterol [14, 63, 70]. Among haemodynamic changes (Figs. 11, 12) increases of intravasal blood pressure seem to be associated with increased prostacyclin formation [266] as does acute ischaemia [159]. In the kidney, the increase of glomerular filtration rate produced by increased oral protein intake in healthy probands is accompanied by a definite stimulation of prostacyclin excretion, though in patients with renal failure prostacyclin stimulation fails to occur despite increased renal filtration performance [49]. Among various groups of drugs, a prostacyclin-stimulating action was demonstrated not only for antihypertensive agents (see Chap. 4.3), but also for pentoxifylline [160, 286] and glyceryl trinitrate [144].

Inhibition of Prostacyclin Synthesis

As with the other eicosanoids, an inhibition of prostacyclin synthesis can be achieved by inhibiting arachidonic acid metabolism with indomethacin, acetylsalicylic acid and meclofenamic acid (Fig. 13). The essentially specific inhibitors of prostacyclin synthetase are β-thromboglobulin [121], tranylcypromine [94] and fatty acid peroxides, especially 15-hydroperoxyarachidonic

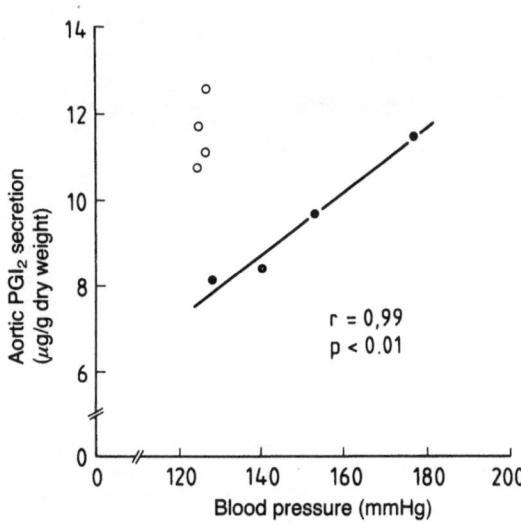

Fig. 11. Relation between mean aortic prostacyclin liberation and mean arterial blood pressure in Dahl salt-resistant (○) and salt-sensitive (●) rats [266]

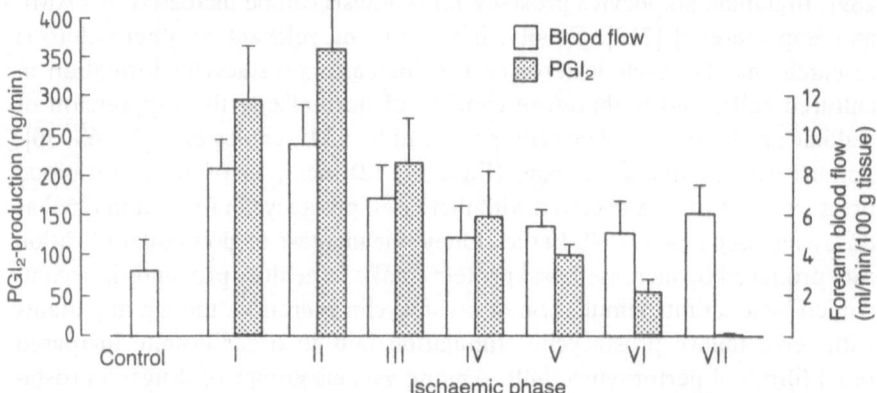

Fig. 12. Stimulation of vascular prostacyclin synthesis in the forearm by ischaemia and its continued exhaustion by repeated ischaemia. The change in forearm blood pressure is shown for comparison ($\bar{x} \pm SD$) [159]

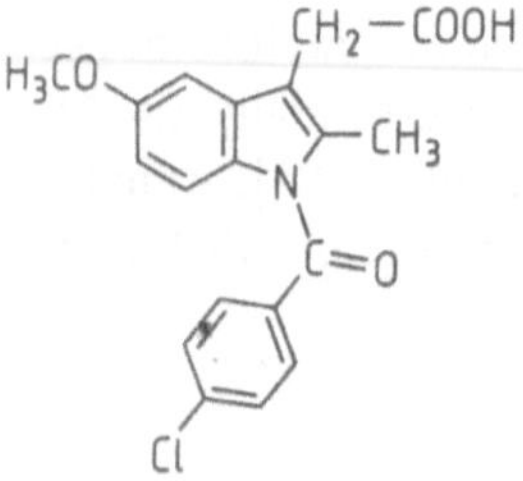

Indomethacin

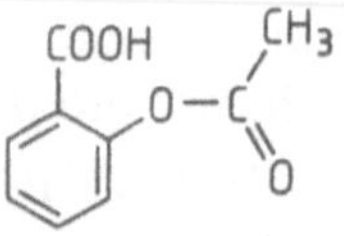

Acetylsalicylic acid

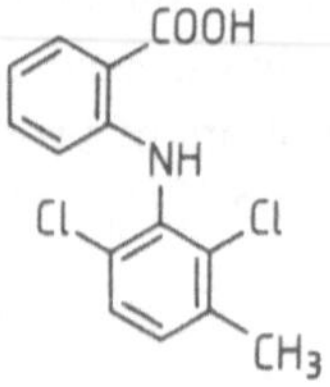

Meclofenamic acid

a Cyclooxygenase inhibitors

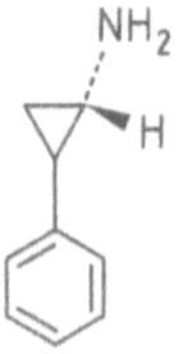

Tranylcypromine

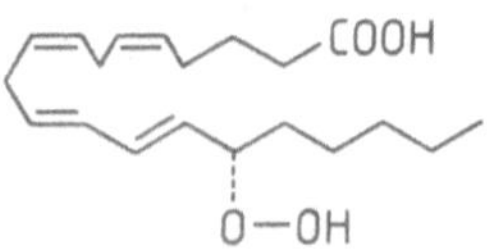

15-hydroperoxy-
arachidonic acid
(15-HPETE)

b Prostacyclin synthetase inhibitors

Fig. 13. a, b. Inhibitors of prostacyclin synthesis

acid (15-HPETE) [106, 169]. Among drugs, glucocorticoids (hydrocortisone) seem able to cause inhibition of prostacyclin synthesis, as demonstrated by short-term experiments in rabbits [171]. Testosterone also leads to a definite reduction in vascular prostacyclin formation [187], whereas estradiol seems to stimulate it [31].

3 Activity Profile of Prostacyclin

3.1 Local Activity Profile

It is very probable that prostacyclin produces its local effects via specific fixation sites as has been demonstrated at least for the platelets and erythrocytes [167, 240]. In the platelets the fixation site for prostacyclin is identical with that for PGE_2, whereas 6-oxo-$PGF_{1\alpha}$ as a breakdown product of prostacyclin does not contract any fixation at this site [289].

Thrombocytic Action
The prostacyclin formed by the endothelium plays a decisive part in the interrelation between vascular endothelium and platelets, in that it antagonizes the action of thromboxane A_2 formed by the platelets (Fig. 14). After their activation the platelets increase their formation of thromboxane A_2, which in turn promotes platelet aggregation and adhesion to the endothelium. At the vessel wall thromboxane A_2 leads to muscular contraction. In the platelets themselves the formation of cAMP is decreased by the liberation of thromboxane, resulting in a secondary increase in the activity of phospholipase A_2. In this way thromboxane A_2 can stimulate its own synthesis rate. On the other hand, even in low concentrations, prostacyclin has an antiaggregatory effect on the thrombocytes (Fig. 15) [193]. In addition, in high concentrations it inhibits platelet adhesion to the endothelium. Correspondingly, in experiments on rats, rabbits and guinea pigs, platelet adhesion to damaged endothelium was clearly correlated with the existing endothelial liberation of prostacyclin (Fig. 16) [263]. Locally, prostacyclin can even break up platelet aggregations and so prevent thromboembolic occlusion of the smallest vessels (capillaries). This is, for instance, particularly important in maintaining the microcirculation in the lungs [174]. Inhibition of prostacyclin formation by hydrocortisone, acetylsalicylic acid or tranylcypromine abolishes all these favourable effects of prostacyclin in vitro and thus leads to increased thrombus formation [132]. In the platelets prostacyclin stimulates the activity of adenylate cyclase [89] and thus reduces the concentration of free calcium in the cells [267]. Via this alteration in free calcium it eventually inhibits the activity of phospholipase A_2 and hence the synthesis of thromboxane A_2.

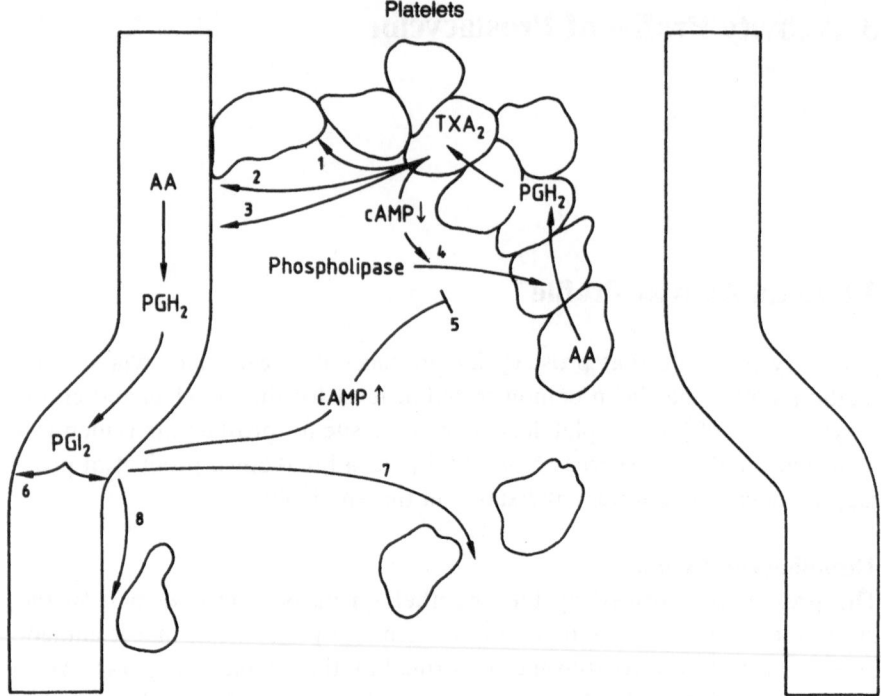

Fig. 14. Interaction between vessels and platelets. The activated platelets predominantly synthesize thromboxane A_2 (*TXA$_2$*) from arachidonic acid, thereby producing (*1*) their aggregation (*2*) their adhesion to the vascular endothelium (*3*) vessel contraction, and (*4*) stimulation of phospholipase A_2. The vascular endothelium synthesizes almost exclusively PGI$_2$ from arachidonic acid (*AA*). This develops an antagonistic action to the thromboxane A_2 of the platelets and (*5*) reduces the activity of phospholipase A_2, (*6*) dilates the vessel, (*7*) prevents platelet aggregation and (*8*) finally also reduces platelet adhesion to the vessel endothelium

Correspondingly, the action of prostacyclin can be markedly increased by the inhibition of cAMP breakdown, for instance by phosphodiesterase inhibitory agents like theophyllin [96, 168, 282], and can be significantly weakened by inhibition of adenylate cyclase activity with 2',5'-dideoxy-adenosine [110]. Prostacyclin produces a marked and direct vasodilatation at the vessel itself. The fluctuation between thrombocytic thromboxane A_2 and endothelial prostacyclin is particularly exciting as the action of prostacyclin suggests a fine-tuned regulation of platelet-endothelial interaction. Immediately after their activation the platelets liberate the cyclooxygenase product PGH$_2$, which can increase prostacyclin synthesis in the endothelium even without stimulation of endogenous endothelial arachidonic acid metabolism [172]. Prostacyclin

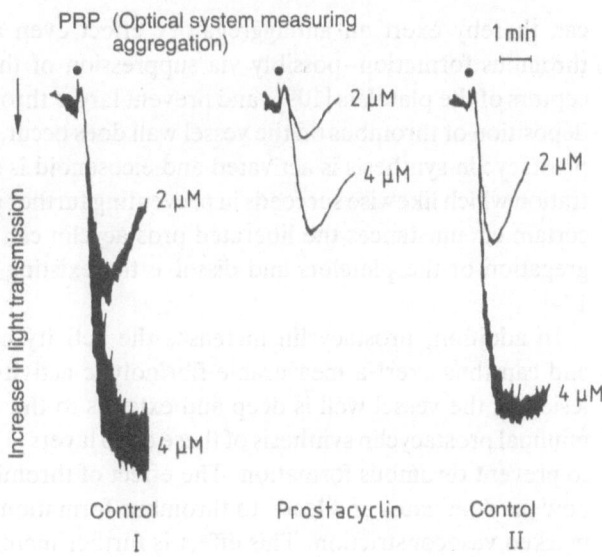

Fig. 15. Inhibitory effect of prostacyclin on ADP-induced aggregation of human thrombocytes. In the *control phases I* and *II* the platelets were incubated only with the solvent. In the *experimental phase prostacyclin* was added to the solvent in a concentration of 8 ng/kg per min for 15 min. In the control phases, ADP in two concentrations (2 and 4 μM) produced a dose-dependent aggregation of the platelets, whereas in the experimental phase there was scarcely any increase in light transmission, and platelet aggregation was largely absent [193]

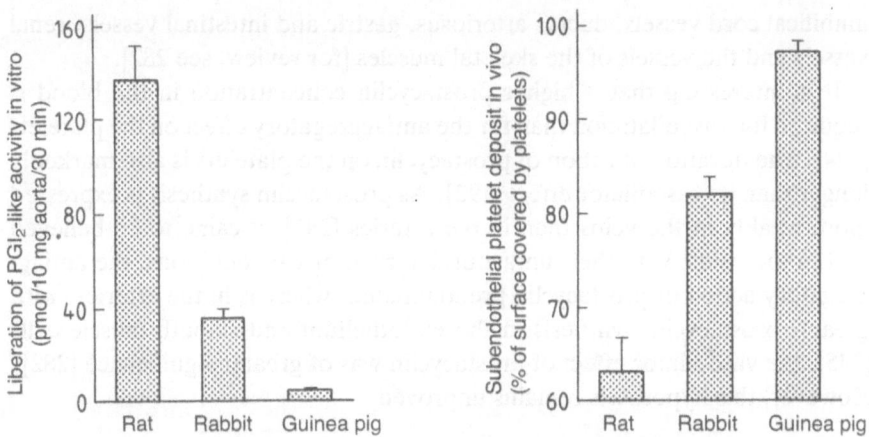

Fig. 16. Inverse relation between aortic prostacyclin synthesis and endothelial platelet adhesion in different animal species after endothelial damage ($\bar{x} \pm$ SEM) [263]

can thereby exert an antiaggregatory effect even at a very early stage of thrombus formation–possibly via suppression of the surface fibrinogen receptors of the platelets [109]–and prevent larger thrombi [4]. If, nevertheless, deposition of thrombus on the vessel wall does occur, endogenous endothelial prostacyclin synthesis is activated and eicosanoid is secreted in high concentration which likewise succeeds in preventing further platelet adhesion. Under certain circumstances the liberated prostacyclin can even bring about disaggregation of the platelets and dissolve the existing microthrombus [96, 97, 174].

In addition, prostacyclin increases the activity of plasminogen activator and can thus exert a measurable fibrinolytic activity [176]. However, if the lesion of the vessel wall is deep and extends to the media or adventitia, the minimal prostacyclin synthesis of these deep layers [170] is no longer adequate to prevent thrombus formation. The effect of thrombocytic thromboxane A_2 now predominates and leads to thrombus formation and adhesion as well as marked vasoconstriction. This effect is further increased by local thromboxane A_2 formation in the adventitial tissue.

Vascular Action

Prostacyclin is classed as one of the most potent vasodilators as yet known in the body. Its effect is approximately 8 times as great as that of PGE_2 and some 100 times greater than that of its breakdown product 6-oxo-$PGF_{1\alpha}$ [6]. Prostacyclin exerts its vasodilator action independently of the nature (artery or vein), size (aorta or capillary) and site (organ) of the vessel by relaxing the smooth muscle of the vessel [174]. The vasodilator action of prostacyclin has so far been demonstrated for the aorta, coronary vessels, pulmonary vessels, umbilical cord vessels, ductus arteriosus, gastric and intestinal vessels, renal vessels and the vessels of the skeletal muscles [for review, see 282].

It is interesting that a higher prostacyclin concentration in the blood is required for vasodilatation than for the antiaggregatory effect on the platelets [174]. The duration of action of prostacyclin on the platelets is also markedly longer than its vasodilator effect [193]. As prostacyclin synthesis is expressed more weakly in the veins than in the arteries [245], it came to be believed that in the veins, with their unfavourable rheological conditions, the antiaggregatory action of prostacyclin predominated, whereas in the arteries, with greater prostacyclin synthesis in the endothelium and smooth muscle cells [245], the vasodilator effect of prostacyclin was of greater significance [282]. However, this hypothesis remains unproved.

Cytoprotective Action

Prostacyclin also appears to exert a so-called "cytoprotective" action, which has been particularly well-investigated for the myocardial cells [242]. Thus it can be observed that during treatment with prostacyclin and its analogues the size of an infarct after experimental ischaemia is smaller than without prostacyclin treatment, and that reperfusion arrhythmias after ischaemia are significantly reduced by prostacyclin, independently of whether the eicosanoid is infused before or during the ischaemic phase [143, 180]. Also, in patients with myocardial infarction, prostacyclin can limit the myocardial destruction and act protectively [113]. The ultimate mechanism of this cardioprotective action is unclear at the present time. On the one hand, the vasodilation and reduced platelet aggregation play a part, but these effects alone do not seem adequate to account for the cytoprotection. Additional effects, such as the inhibition of chemotaxis and the activation of neutrophil leucocytes [287] as well as stabilization of their lysosomal membranes [143] appear to be necessary to explain the cellular action of prostacyclin. Evidence for such a lysosomal effect of prostacyclin is provided by findings in cells of the liver and gastric mucosa and nerve cells which show that after toxic damage to these cells prostacyclin can significantly reduce the activity of lysosomal hydrolases of migrant granulocytes [16, 26, 28, 289]. Further investigations are required for more complete elucidation of the so-called "cytoprotective" action of prostacyclin and to arrive at definite conclusions.

Antiatherogenic Action

Atherosclerotic lesions of the human aorta are marked by lipid deposits. The cholesterol esters are the main components of these lipids [36]. Prostacyclin is capable of counteracting the accumulation of cholesterol esters [103, 104, 105]. The mechanism by which prostacyclin removes the cholesterol esters from the smooth muscle cells of the aortic wall has been exhaustively studied in the rabbit aorta (Fig. 17) [105]. Prostacyclin stimulates the intracellular adenylate cyclase and thus increases the cell content of cAMP. The cAMP in its turn stimulates the breakdown of the cholesterol esters by activating cholesterol ester hydrolase. The cholesterol so formed is then eliminated from the cell into the extracellular space by means of a sterol carrier protein, e.g. high density lipoprotein (HDL). The same effect, namely the reduction of the intracellular content of cholesterol esters, can also be demonstrated for the prostacyclin analogue, carbacyclin [199]. This cellular action of prostacyclin is possibly of special significance in the pathogenesis of atherosclerosis and its therapeutic management. When atherosclerosis is clinically obvious, the vascular tissue is no longer capable of adequately forming prostacyclin [138]. On the basis of the investigations discussed here, this local deficiency

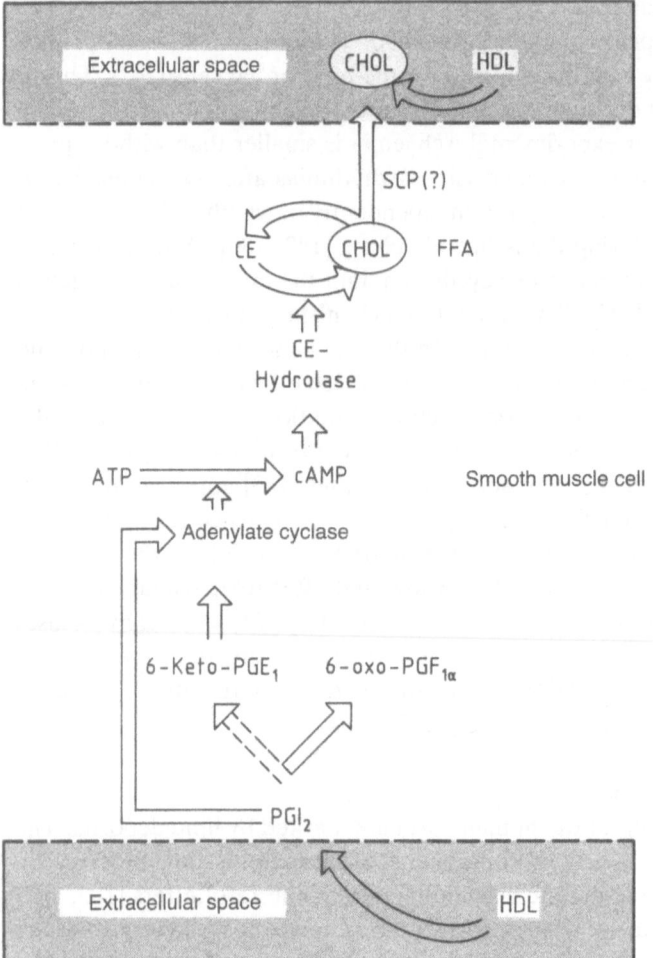

Fig. 17. Hypothetical model of prostacyclin action on cholesterol metabolism in smooth muscle of vessel wall (after Hajjar). By forming cAMP, prostacyclin activates cholesterol ester (*CE*) hydrolase to liberate cholesterol (*CHOL*), which is then transported out of the cell by a sterol carrier protein (*SCP*) [104, 105]

in prostacyclin could result in the vascular tissue no longer being capable of effectively counteracting further deposition of cholesterol esters, so that the atheromatosis would advance rapidly. On the other hand, it might be theorized that the employment in clinical treatment of prostacyclin or its analogues could lead to a regression of lipid deposition and improvement in the atherosclerotic clinical picture. However, confirmation of this hypothesis in vivo is

24

still lacking and we must wait and see whether therapeutic consequences can be derived from these findings.

3.2 Action on Circulatory Regulation

Regulation of Systemic Circulation
In nearly all species prostacyclin induces a fall in systemic blood pressure. As prostacyclin does not undergo any pulmonary metabolism [6], its blood pressure-reducing effect is independent of the mode of administration, which means that it exerts the same effect on the circulation whether infused intravenously or intraarterially. The reduction of blood pressure by prostacyclin is dose dependent and begins in the rat with an infusion rate of about 2 μg/ kg per min [6] and in humans at about 2 ng/kg per min [17]. In the anaesthetized rat with the vascular system precontracted by angiotensin II, it can be shown that the vasodilatation produced by prostacyclin develops immediately – even within the first minute – and has already completely disappeared again after 10 – 15 min (Fig. 18) [231]. The actual fall in blood pressure is due entirely to a strictly dose-dependent reduction of the total vascular resistance (Fig. 19) [223]. There is a reflex rise in the heart rate and a minor increase of cardiac output and the stroke volume index [17, 32]. The fall in total vascular resistance is based on a decline of resistance in all vascular regions as prostacyclin acts similarly in all vascular areas. Given intravenously, prostacyclin exerts an effect on the human systemic circulation approximately 20 times greater than that of PGE_2, which acts on the circulation only in doses of about 40 ng/kg per min [235]. The difference in the action of the two substances on the blood pressure is explained by their differing pulmonary metabolism. PGE_2 is 95 % inactivated by lung passage [175], whereas prostacyclin remains unaffected. Under certain circumstances, with low infusion rates, prostacyclin produces only an erythema of the skin of the face and hands. With increased dosage it develops a dilatation of the resistant systemic vessels with consequent fall in blood pressure, more marked for the diastolic than for the systolic pressure. In high doses prostacyclin produces headaches of vascular origin and, due to excessive fall in blood pressure, tachycardia, nausea, pallor and unrest. All these studies show that exogenous prostacyclin can exert a marked vasodepressor action. However, these pharmacological studies do not allow the conclusion that prostacyclin is fundamentally involved in blood pressure regulation. Numerous studies which have demonstrated prostacyclin in the circulation were based on measurement of the stable, but biologically inactive breakdown product, 6-oxo-$PGF_{1\alpha}$. However, no conclusions may be drawn from this metabolite as to the amount of circulating active prostacyclin, as

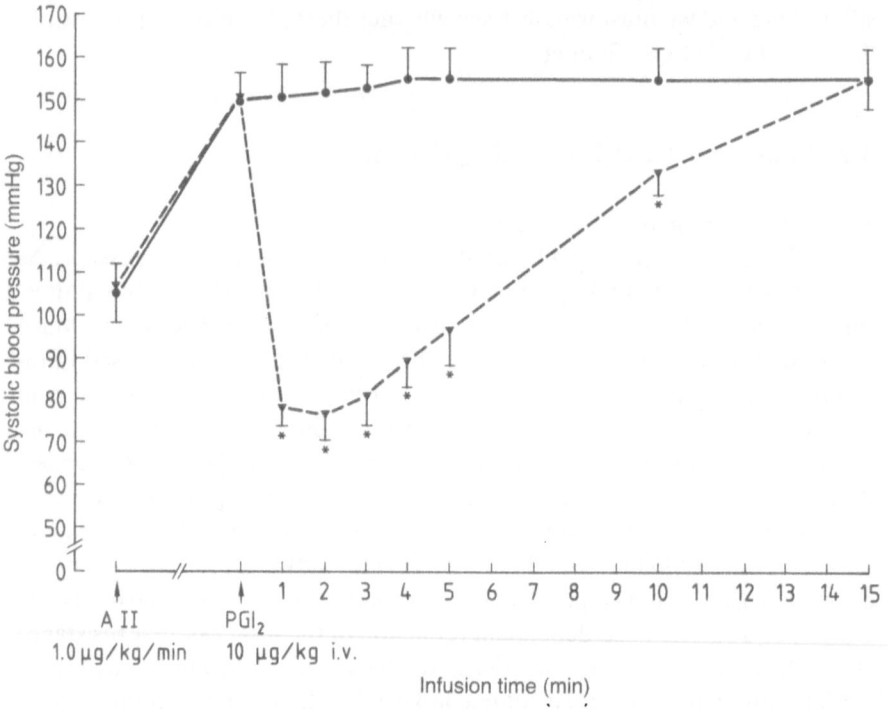

Fig. 18. Fall in systolic blood pressure after intravenous injection of prostacyclin in anaesthetized rats during blood pressure elevation induced by angiotensin II (A II). (●——●, control group, $n = 5$; ▼- - -▼, PGI$_2$ group, $n = 5$; $\bar{x} \pm$ SEM; * $P < 0.05$) [231]

this may equally well arise directly from the vascular tissue compartment. In individual cases, however, it is possible to directly demonstrate circulating amounts of prostacyclin which are capable of exerting biological activities [84, 100]. Indirect evidence of the involvement of the prostaglandins, also including prostacyclin, are provided by studies with inhibition of prostaglandin synthesis by indomethacin, or with stimulation of endogenous prostaglandin synthesis by oral administration of arachidonic acid precursors or polyunsaturated fatty acids.

Fig. 20. Changes in mean systemic blood pressure, systemic total resistance and renal resistance under *basal* conditions and after intravenous administration of 50 mg indomethacin (*Indo*). ($\bar{x} \pm$ SEM; ** $P < 0.01$; *** $P < 0.001$) [191]

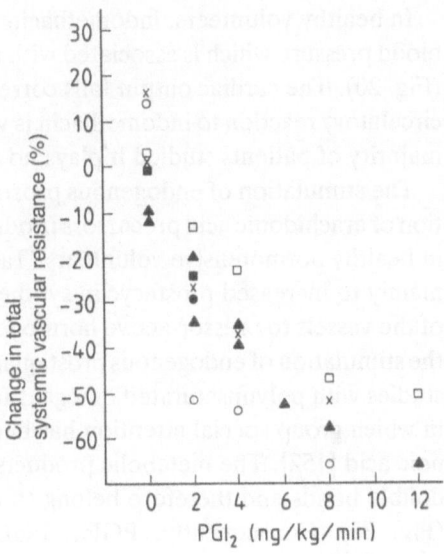

Fig. 19. Dose-dependent influence of intravenously administered prostacy-clin (*PGI₂*) on total systemic vascular resistance. The percentage changes are shown compared with the control group. The null dose stands for the effect of the glycine buffer as solvent. *Each symbol* stands for one patient [223]

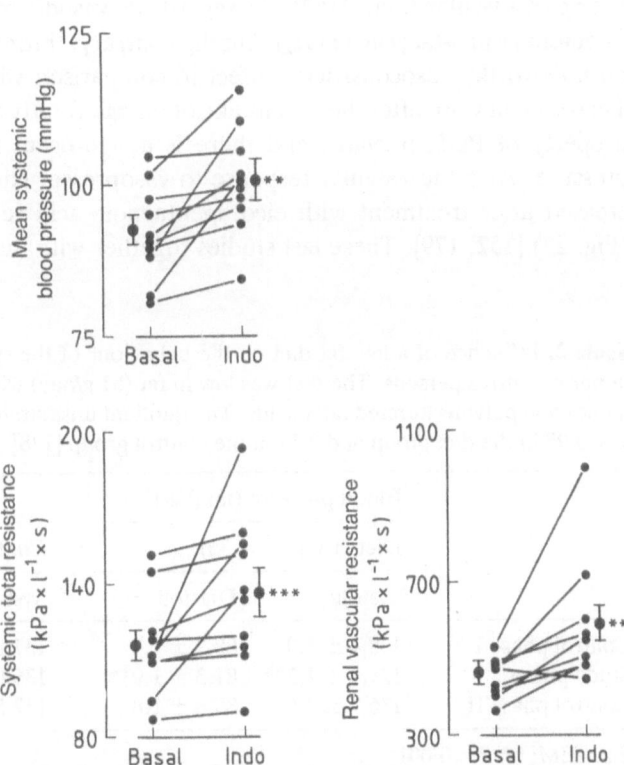

Fig. 20

In healthy volunteers, indomethacin [191] leads to a minor rise in systemic blood pressure which is associated with an increase in total vascular resistance (Fig. 20). The cardiac output falls correspondingly [270, 290]. The individual circulatory reaction to indomethacin is very variable, but in the overwhelming majority of patients studied it plays no noteworthy part in clinical routine.

The stimulation of endogenous prostaglandin synthesis by oral administration of arachidonic acid precursors produces a significant fall in blood pressure in healthy normotensive volunteers (Table 2) [212], which is to be attributed mainly to increased prostacyclin synthesis (Fig. 10) [60]. Also, the response of the vessels to pressor-active hormones such as angiotensin II is reduced by the stimulation of endogenous prostaglandins (Fig. 21) [233]. However, recent studies with polyunsaturated omega-3-fatty acids are particularly interesting, in which group special attention has been paid to the effect of eicosapentaenoic acid [152]. The metabolic products of eicosapentaenoic acid have three double bonds and therefore belong to the third series of the prostaglandins (Fig. 22). Consequently, PGE_3, PGD_3, PGI_3 and thromboxane A_3 are formed. Under certain conditions the vascular prostaglandin PGI_3 and thrombocytic thromboxane A_3 as its antagonist are of special importance in the fine tuning of vascular tonus [152]. As regards its vasodilator effect, PGI_3 is just as potent as prostacyclin (PGI_2). On the contrary, thromboxane A_3 possesses no noteworthy vasoconstrictor effect in comparison with thromboxane A_2. Therefore in vivo, after the oral intake of omega-3-fatty acids, the vasodilator property of PGI_3 prevails, and there is a significant fall in resting blood pressure. Also the vascular response to vasopressor stimuli is markedly decreased after treatment with eicosapentaenoic acid (e.g. as cod-liver oil), (Fig. 23) [152, 179]. These last studies together with the findings after indo-

Table 2. Influence of a low fat diet on the behaviour of the systemic blood pressure in normotensive persons. The diet was low in fat (51 g/day) with a high proportion of mono- and polyunsaturated fatty acids. The quotient unsaturated/saturated fatty acids was 0.98 in the diet group and 0.17 in the control group [128]

| | Blood pressure (mmHg) | | | |
| | Diet group ($n = 35$) | | Control group ($n = 38$) | |
	Systolic	Diastolic	Systolic	Diastolic
Control phase I	$138,4 \pm 3,0$	$88,9 \pm 1,9$	$137,8 \pm 2,0$	$89,3 \pm 1,5$
Study phase	$129,5 \pm 2,2**$	$81,3 \pm 1,0**$	$136,0 \pm 2,1$	$86,9 \pm 1,5$
Control phase II	$136,7 \pm 2,6$	$85,3 \pm 1,8$	$137,5 \pm 2,2$	$87,6 \pm 1,5$

$\bar{x} \pm$ SEM; ** $P < 0.001$

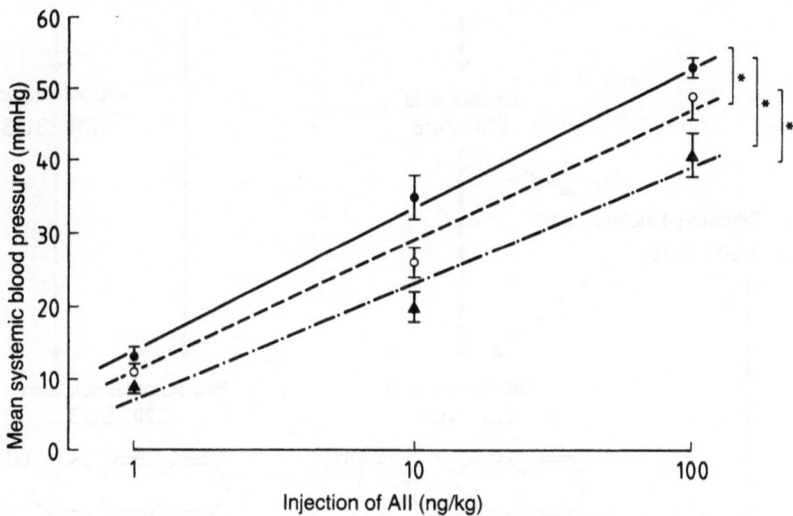

Fig. 21. Effect of olive oil and evening primrose oil on the increased blood pressure induced in anaesthetized rats by the intravenous administration of angiotensin II (*A II*). (•——•, controls; ○–––○, olive oil 1 ml/day po for 90 days; ▲–·–▲, evening primrose oil 1 ml/day po for 90 days ($\bar{x} \pm$ SEM; $P < 0.05$) [233]

methacin suggest that under normal conditions, prostacyclin and thromboxane A_2 are reciprocally involved in the fine adjustment of systemic blood pressure and that a disturbance of their biological equilibrium is immediately expressed as a sizeable change in blood pressure.

Renal Circulatory Regulation

Basal renal perfusion seems from animal experimental studies [260] not to be directly dependent on prostaglandin and therefore not on prostacyclin synthesis, as indomethacin produces no change in basal renal perfusion in the unanaesthetized dog (Fig. 21) [233]. Yet, on the other hand, there is adequate evidence from studies in unanaesthetized rabbits and healthy probands that indomethacin can increase the basal vascular resistance of the kidney (Fig. 20) [13, 191]. However, the conditions are different and more uniform in acute renal damage and nervous (sympathetic) renal stresses [161, 260]. Here there is an intrarenal stimulation of prostacyclin, and under these conditions indomethacin is capable of restructing renal perfusion. Stimulation of intrarenal prostaglandin synthesis by arachidonic acid or bradykinin infusion produces an increased perfusion of the renal medulla and juxtamedullary cortex [161, 282]. In these tissue regions vascular prostacyclin synthesis predominates over the other vasoconstrictor prostaglandins. Thus, prostacyclin leads via

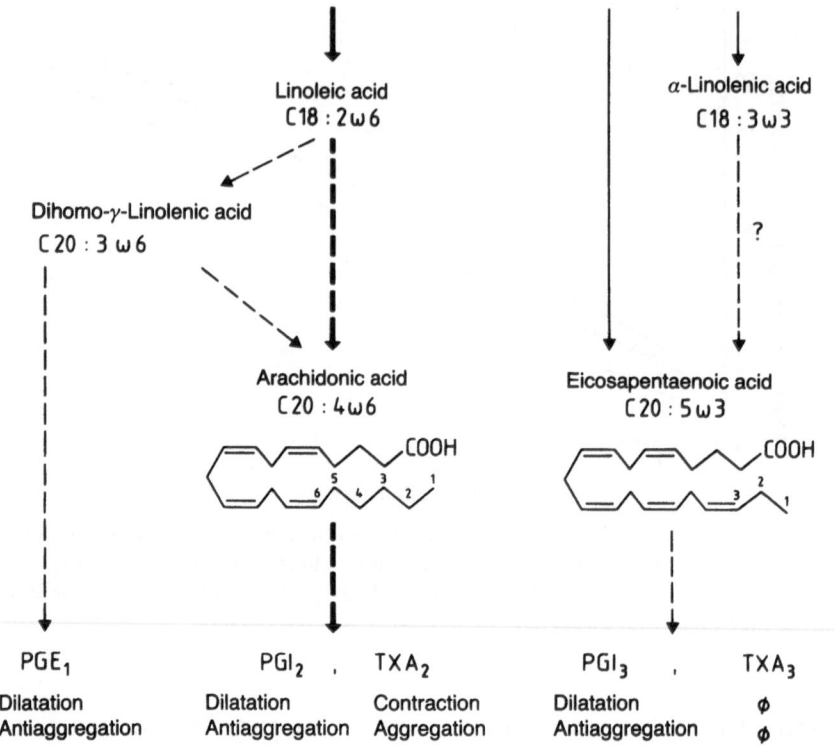

Fig. 22. Metabolism of polyunsaturated fatty acids. The omega-6-fatty acids are a constitutent of the standard western diet; the omega-3-fatty acids, especially eicosapentaenoic acid, predominate in certain marine animals. Specifically in humans, the omega-3- and omega-6-fatty acids are not interconvertible [152]

local vasodilatation to the described redistribution of the renal circulation. In the autoregulation of the kidney the locally formed prostacyclin appears to exert a counter-regulatory function against the vasopressor hormones since it can markedly reduce the vasoconstrictor effect of the activated sympathetic nervous system and of the stimulated renin-angiotensin system [161]. Prostacyclin increases renal sodium excretion and diuresis, even without influencing the glomerular filtration rate [101]. As it is present almost exclusively in the renal vessels and not in the tubular endothelium [234], the influence of prostacyclin on diuresis and natriuresis must be attributed mainly to vascular changes [54]. The redistribution of blood in favour of the marrow and inner cortex may play a decisive role here. In vitro studies suggest that a direct tubular action of prostacyclin is rather unlikely [282].

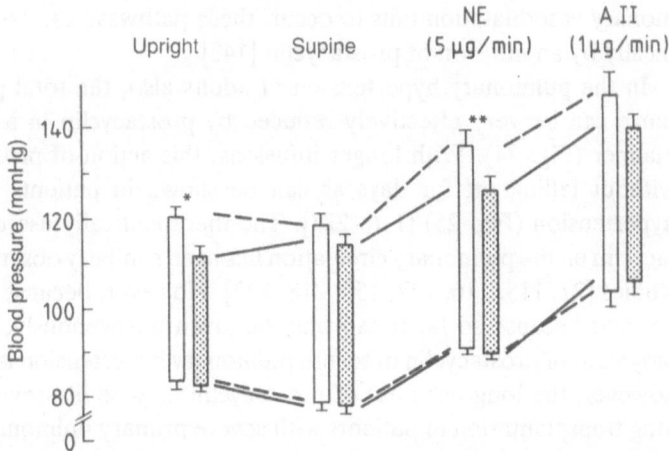

		NE	A II
Upright	Supine	(5 µg/min)	(1µg/min)

Fig. 23. Change in basic standing and lying blood pressure and its reaction to nor-epinephrine (*NE*) and angiotensin II (*A II*) produced by a 25-day diet supplemented by cod-liver oil. (*Upper end of bars*, systolic blood pressure; *lower end of bars*, diastolic blood pressure; *open bars*, control group, $n = 8$; *stippled bars*, cod-liver oil diet, $n = 8$; $\bar{x} \pm$ SEM; * $P < 0.05$; ** $P < 0.01$) [152]

It is very probable that the renal effects of prostacyclin are based only on the locally formed agent since the prostacyclin concentrations necessary for the vasodilatation and natriuresis are markedly higher (tenfold in the dog) than the normal concentrations of prostacyclin in the circulating blood [54].

Pulmonary Circulatory Regulation

Prostacyclin plays an important part in the vessels of the pulmonary circulation since it is necessary for maintaining perfusion in the lung periphery. It not only regulates vascular dilatation, but also prevents a thrombotic status in the lung capillaries when blood flow is slow and can rapidly redissolve any clumped microthrombi [38]. The significance of prostacyclin for the pulmonary circulation is best demonstrated in the lungs of the newborn. Until parturition prostacyclin is the chief product of cyclooxygenase metabolism in the ductus arteriosus [202, 261]. Here, together with the simultaneously synthesized PGE_2, it keeps the vessel patent and thus provides for the intact fetal circulation. Accordingly, the inhibition of cyclooxygenase metabolism by indomethacin leads to rapid closure of the ductus [238, 250]. After parturition, intrapulmonary prostacyclin synthesis is stimulated by hypoxia [159] and thus most probably leads to the opening up of the circulatory pathways of the lung that have been closed up to this time [38]. If post-partum pulmonary vasodilatation fails to occur, these pathways can be opened iatrogenically by an infusion of prostacyclin [148].

In the pulmonary hypertension of adults also, the total pulmonary resistance can be very effectively reduced by prostacyclin in a dose-dependent manner (Fig. 24). With longer infusions, this action of prostacyclin persists without falling off for days as can be shown in patients with pulmonary hypertension (Fig. 25) [116, 223]. The therapeutically useful effect of prostacyclin on the pulmonary circulation has been similarly observed in numerous studies [27, 115, 116, 127, 150, 218, 223]. However, because of its short half-life and because so far it can only be given intravenously, the clinical employment of prostacyclin in severe pulmonary hypertension is not practicable; however, the long-term use of prostacyclin may be life-saving before heart-lung transplantation in patients with severe primary pulmonary hypertension [150]. Despite the numerous clinical studies and the reproducible therapeutic effect, it is still unclear whether primary or secondary pulmonary hypertension can be attributed to an endogenous deficiency of pulmonary prostacyclin. It would seem that further extensive studies are urgently required to clarify the pathogenetic importance of prostacyclin in pulmonary hypertension.

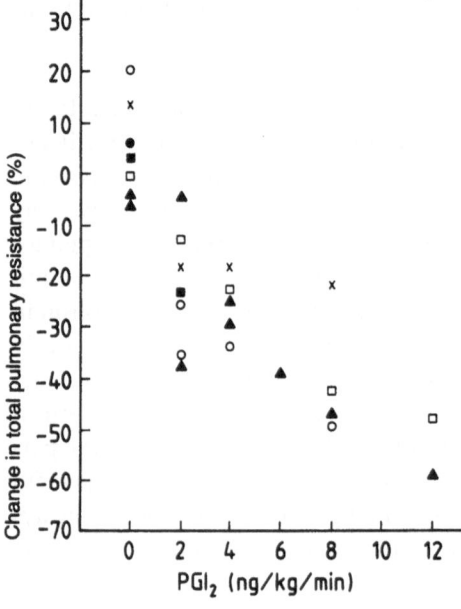

Fig. 24. Dose-dependent influence of intravenously administered prostacyclin (PGI_2) on total pulmonary resistance. The percentage changes are shown in comparison with the control group. The null dose stands for the effect of the glycine buffer as solvent. *Each symbol* stands for one patient [223]

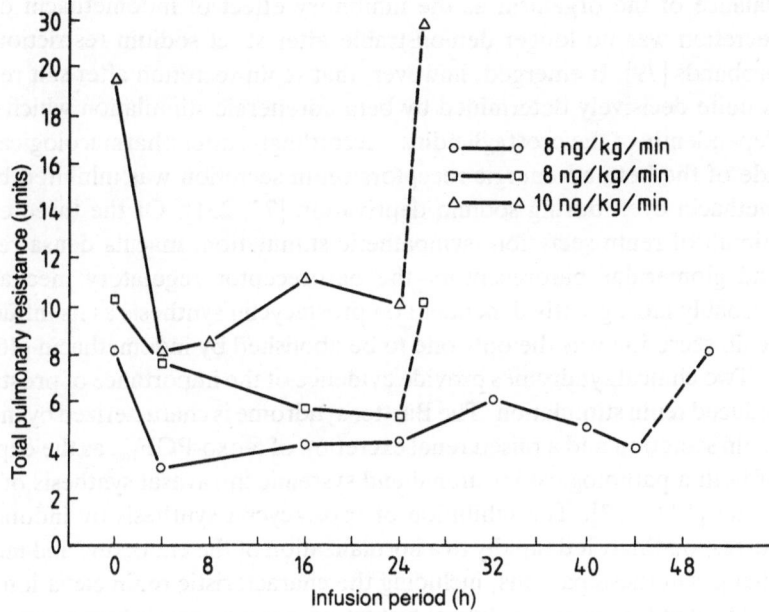

Fig. 25. Reduction of total pulmonary resistance by prostacyclin in three patients with pulmonary hypertension. The *dotted line* shows the prompt recurrent increase in pulmonary vascular resistance after termination of prostacyclin infusion [223]

3.3 Interference with Other Vasoactive Hormones

Renin-Angiotensin System

According to recent studies, among the vascular prostaglandins it is vascular prostacyclin that has the most effective action on the renal renin secretion [79, 231]. It has been shown in vitro that renin secretion by the renal cortical tissue can be stimulated by prostacyclin, whereas PGE_2 is without effect [206, 280, 293]. Also, renin secretion in the isolated perfused kidney is stimulated by prostacyclin [194]. Moreover, it was also shown in this study that prostacyclin not only promotes renin secretion, but also the activation of inactive to active renin (Fig. 26). Stimulation of renin secretion was also possible with arachidonic acid, whereas inhibition of prostaglandin synthesis by indomethacin led to a regression of renin secretion [76, 137, 273, 285, 293]. In these experiments prostacyclin proved equipotent to isoproterenol in its molar effect. Only in very few studies did prostacyclin have no stimulating effect on renin liberation comparable to its analogue iloprost [301]. Initially, the stimulation of renin by the prostaglandins seemed dependent on the sodium balance of the organism as the inhibitory effect of indomethacin on renin secretion was no longer demonstrable after strict sodium restriction in the probands [79]. It emerged, however, that renin secretion after salt reduction is quite decisively determined by beta-adrenergic stimulation which acts independently of the prostaglandins. Accordingly, after pharmacological blockade of the beta-adrenergic receptors renin secretion was inhibited by indomethacin even during sodium deprivation [77, 231]. Of the three essential stimuli of renin secretion–sympathetic stimulation, macula densa receptors and glomerular baroreceptors–the baroreceptor regulatory mechanism is probably most greatly dependent on prostacyclin synthesis as its influence on renin secretion was the only one to be abolished by indomethacin [46].

Two clinical syndromes provide evidence of the importance of prostacyclin-induced renin stimulation. The Bartter syndrome is characterized by increased renin secretion and a raised renal excretion of 6-oxo-PGF$_{1\alpha}$, as the expression of both a pathological intrarenal and systemic intravasal synthesis of prostacyclin [100, 222]. The inhibition of prostacyclin synthesis by indomethacin correspondingly led rapidly to a normalization of the endocrine and metabolic changes in these patients, including the characteristic renin elevation [272].

The conditions in the clinical picture of hyporeninemic hypoaldosteronism are exactly the opposite. Here the essential cause of the endocrine and

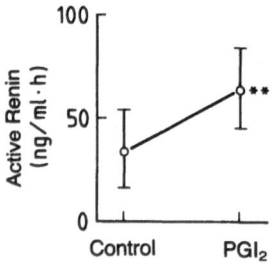

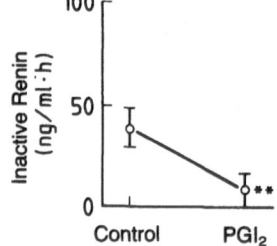

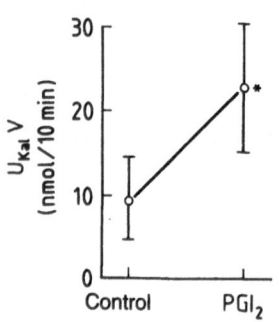

Fig. 26. Influence of prostacyclin infusion on the excretion of kallikrein in the urine ($U_{Kal}V$) and on the activity of active and inactive renin in the plasma

($\bar{x} \pm$ SEM; * $P < 0.05$; ** $P < 0.01$) [194]

metabolic changes in these patients was revealed as a deficiency of endogenous prostacyclin with a reduced response to stimulation [173]. Therefore the substitution of prostacyclin compensates for the lack of the endogenous eicosanoid and leads to a normalization of all the pathological changes and also to a normalization of the previously suppressed renin and aldosterone activity [295].

There is a close interrelation between the renin-angiotensin system and prostacyclin. Thus, for its part, active renin can stimulate prostacyclin synthesis via the formation of angiotensin II [103, 181, 239]. This angiotensin II effect, though not described by every author [182], is now undisputed and is interpreted as an important control of the vascular effect of angiotensin II [164]. Prostacyclin is formed in the cortical vessels and also in the afferent arterioles of the glomeruli and can antagonize the vasoconstriction produced by angiotensin II. In this way the kidney is able to protect itself from the detrimental action of the renin-angiotensin system even when the latter is excessively stimulated, as in hypovolemia or renal artery stenosis, and to maintain renal function, especially glomerular filtration [163, 164]. Indirect evidence as to the antagonism of the prostaglandins as well as prostacyclin to angiotensin II is provided by studies showing that after pretreatment with indomethacin the vasopressor effect of angiotensin II is more pronounced [189, 228, 273]. It is a particularly interesting finding that acetylsalicylic acid in high dosage acts similarly to indomethacin, though in lower dosage the action of angiotensin II is markedly weakened [228]. These two different effects of acetylsalicylic acid can be explained by two different modes of action of this substance. In high dosage prostaglandin synthesis is globally inhibited, as also the vascular formation of prostacyclin. However, in low doses (80 mg) prostaglandin synthesis is still maintained; however, there occurs a shift of the thromboxane/prostacyclin ratio in favour of prostacyclin as acetylsalicylic acid in these low doses inhibits only the synthesis of thromboxane A_2 in the platelets [107, 211].

Kallikrein-Kinin System
Studies in the isolated perfused rat's kidney show that renal kallikrein secretion in the urine and in the venous side of the circulation is stimulated by renal prostaglandins [275]. Thus, perfusion of the kidney with a medium containing arachidonic acid increases the outflow of kallikrein both in the venous effluent and the urine of the kidney. This stimulating action of arachidonic acid was completely inhibited by indomethacin. Further differentiation of this global effect of arachidonic acid was not obtained in this study, so that it is impossible on the basis of these data to distinguish whether the kallikrein stimulation is produced by PGE_2 or prostacyclin.

At present, the findings as to the influence of prostacyclin on renal kalli-krein activity are few and contradictory. Thus, in short-term experiments (up to 3 days; Fig. 26) an increase in the urinary excretion of kallikrein after prostacyclin infusion was observed which was always associated with a marked increase in diuresis and natriuresis [35, 194, 208, 301].

However, in these studies it is ultimately undecided whether the increased kallikrein excretion is related to a specific effect of prostacyclin or to a nonspecific diuretic effect. Thus, in numerous studies of the kallikrein-kinin system it was shown that every increase in diuresis is initially associated with

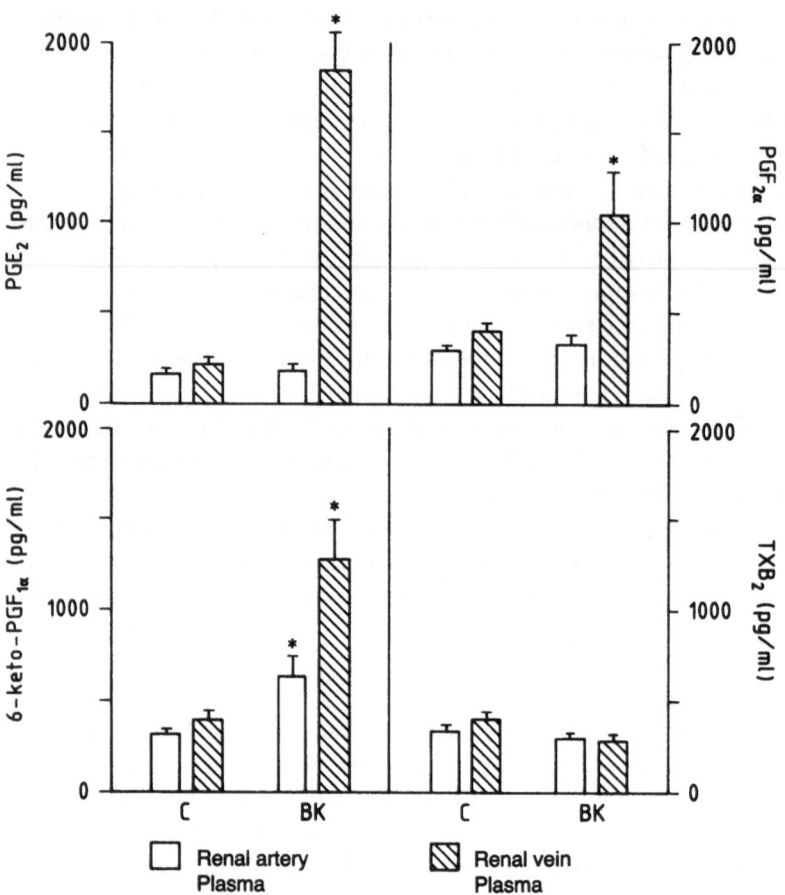

Fig. 27. Concentrations of prostaglandin E_2 (PGE_2), prostaglandin $F_{2\alpha}$ ($PGF_{2\alpha}$), 6-keto-prostaglandin $F_{1\alpha}$ ($PGF_{1\alpha}$) and thromboxane B_2 (TXB_2) in the blood of the renal artery and vein in anaesthetized dogs under basal conditions (C) and after bradykinin infusion (BK) ($\bar{x} \pm$ SEM; $*$ $P < 0.05$) [136]

an increase in renal kallikrein excretion [19]. An argument for a nonspecific reaction of the renal kallikrein in the short-term experiments is provided by the findings of another study in which, contrary to the above-mentioned studies, no stimulation of kallikrein excretion in the urine by prostacyclin can be observed when diuresis is only slightly increased [68].

While the influence of the prostaglandins on the kallikrein-kinin system is still dubious, there is no doubt that the kinins and especially bradykinin can induce a striking stimulation of prostaglandin synthesis, and this not only in the vascular endothelia (prostacyclin), but also in the kidney, the adipocytes, heart cells, ileal mucosa, fibroblasts and nerve cells [7, 44, 117, 119, 195, 259]. The stimulation of prostaglandin synthesis by kinins is based on an increased activity of phospholipase A_2 and can be completely abolished by mepacrine and indomethacin [40, 217, 271]. The activation of phospholipase A_2 is revealed as calcium dependent and can be modified by changes in intracellular calmodulin or calcium content [294]. An increased intracellular concentration of these substances enhances the effect of kinins on prostaglandin synthesis and a fall in their concentration weakens the kinin effect. Whether changes in the intracellular concentration of cAMP have an additional effect on kinin action or even mediate this remains an open question.

Finally, bradykinin can stimulate all the eicosanoids. So far reproducible results exist for PGE_1, PGE_2, PGF_{2a}, PGI_2 and thromboxane A_2 [7, 40, 44, 117, 162, 213]. Interesting findings were obtained in the dog after intraarterial infusion of bradykinin [196]. In this study bradykinin led to a stimulation of renal synthesis of PGE_2 and prostacyclin, but without any influence on thromboxane synthesis (Fig. 27). An interesting additional finding was an isolated increase in prostacyclin in the arterial blood. Two possible causal mechanisms exist: either an additional prostacyclin stimulation in the systemic circulation or a systemic accumulation of prostacyclin liberated by the kidney due to the well-known absence of pulmonary prostacyclin clearance.

Catecholamines

An influence of prostacyclin on the catecholamines in the blood is not confirmed at the present time. An increase of the catecholamines in the blood is certainly obtained with high doses of prostacyclin, but this increase is nonspecific and based only on the marked fall in systemic blood pressure. In a 3-day study with the prostacyclin analogue iloprost [301] no statistically significant change in catecholamine concentrations in the blood was detected, despite a moderate fall in blood pressure. More exhaustive studies are currently lacking, so that the influence of prostacyclin on the catecholamines remains uncertain. The catecholamines adrenaline and noradrenaline themselves have no noteworthy influence on vascular prostacyclin synthesis, as demonstrated by in vivo studies in the dog [181] and in vitro in the cells of the smooth muscle of the vessels [109]. A study in healthy volunteers showed that renal prostacyclin excretion is stimulated by noradrenaline [182], an effect which was completely abolished by blockade of the α-adrenergic receptors with phenoxybenzamine. However, this observation must be of limited importance as in this study [182] noradrenaline administration led to a marked increase in diuresis, so that other renal mechanisms may have been responsible for the increased excretion of prostacyclin and its metabolites.

Antidiuretic Hormone

The antidiuretic hormone (ADH), also known as arginine-vasopressin, acts by retaining water in the collecting duct of the renal nephron and by a vasoconstrictor action on the arterial vessels of the circulation. Both effects of ADH can be markedly diminished by prostaglandins. Thus its renal action is largely antagonized by prostaglandin E_2 [54] and also the vasopressor properties of ADH are very probably diminished by the vascular prostaglandins. Thus, it has been observed that the so-called vascular "ADH tachyphylaxis" (rapid loss of activity during long-term infusion) can be completely abolished by pretreatment with indomethacin, since, with prostaglandin synthesis inhibited, the vasopressor effect of ADH can be maintained undiminished over a longer infusion period [85]. As to whether prostacyclin has a specific influence on the renal or vascular action of ADH, there are at present no reliable data.

Arginine-vasopressin itself stimulates prostacyclin synthesis in the kidney and vessels [109, 147, 182]. This effect is dose dependent and more marked in the cells of the vascular smooth muscle than that of angiotensin II [109]. In our present state of knowledge, this increased vascular prostacyclin liberation seems to counteract the vasopressor action of ADH and to produce the so-called "ADH tachyphylaxis". Lysine-vasopressin has a similar effect on prostacyclin synthesis, whereas the influence of the nonvasoactive analogue desamino-D-arginine-vasopressin (dDAVP) is incomparably lower [109, 182]. These studies suggest that the vasopressor effect of ADH is necessary to trigger the stimulation of vascular prostacyclin formation.

4 The Significance of Prostacyclin in Hypertension

4.1 Experimental Hypertension

Spontaneous Hypertension in the Animal Model

The cause of spontaneous hypertension in the rat is still not conclusively explained. In addition to the increased activities of vasopressor hormones, a reduced activity of vasodepressor factors has also been proposed as causal. Among the prostaglandins with a vasodepressor effect, prostacyclin, as the main vascular prostaglandin, probably plays the leading part in blood pressure regulation. Whether it exerts its action locally on the vessel or also systemically in the circulation is still unclear. Locally, prostacyclin synthesis appears to be increased in spontaneously hypertensive rats. In vitro studies (Fig. 28) regularly showed increased aortic prostacyclin formation in the spontaneously hypertensive animals compared with normotensive Wistar rats [20, 197, 204]. The formation of thromboxane A_2 was also increased in these animals (Table 3) [39], so that the suspicion arises that the stimulation of prostacyclin may possibly be of a reactive nature to the change in thromboxane metabolism. In spontaneously hypertensive rats of the "stroke-prone" strain, aortic prostacyclin synthesis was equally increased in both subgroups, the "stroke-prone" and the "stroke-resistant" rats. A fall in aortic prostacyclin synthesis

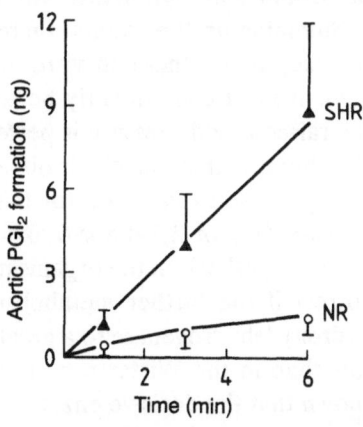

Fig. 28. Liberation of prostacyclin from aortic rings in normotensive (*NR*) and spontaneously hypertensive (*SHR*) rats as a function of incubation time ($\bar{x} \pm$ SEM) [204]

Table 3. Concentration of thromboxane B_2 in serum and excretion of 6-oxo-PGF $_{1\alpha}$ in the urine of spontaneously hypertensive rats and normotensive Wistar-Kyoto rats on a standard diet with hydrogenated coconut oil and sodium salt or water. Values are means with mean deviation of means [31]

Strain	Diet	n	Serum-thromboxane B_2 (ng/ml)	Urinary 6-oxo-PGF$_{1\alpha}$ (ng/24 h)
SHR	HCO/salt	8	533 ± 40*	42,1 ± 5,3*
	HCO/water	9	454 ± 27*	30,3 ± 3,6*
WKY	HCO/salt	8	333 ± 29	67,6 ± 5,1
	HCO/water	6	250 ± 34	52,8 ± 6,4

SHR, spontaneously hypertensive rats; WKY, Wistar-Kyoto rats; HCO, hydrogenated coconut oil
$\bar{x}$ ± SEM; * $P < 0.05$

was observed in some rats of the "stroke-prone" strain only with the development of the actual stroke [197]. This finding is possibly explained by the marked atherosclerotic vascular changes in these animals, for with increasing atherosclerosis of the vessels their rate of prostacyclin synthesis continuously declines [47, 95, 139].

Possibly, renal prostacyclin excretion reflects not only the rate of prostacyclin synthesis in the kidney, but also that of the entire vascular system of the organism. It is basally low in the spontaneously hypertensive rats (Table 3) and can be stimulated only inadequately by salt loading of the diet (Fig. 29) [39, 158]. Also, the stimulation of prostacyclin synthesis by the inhibition of thromboxane metabolism, as is normally observed [155], is not demonstrable in spontaneously hypertensive rats, despite effective inhibition of thromboxane synthetase with the specific inhibitor UK 38,485 [264].

Summing up the results, there is a striking discrepancy between vascular prostacyclin synthesis in vitro and the renal excretion of its metabolites in vivo. It must consequently be surmised that the vascular tissue exposed to the raised blood pressure is perfectly capable of forming increased prostacyclin, but that this capacity is obviously not involved in the circulation in vivo.

A possible explanation for this discrepancy could be that the metabolites 6-oxo-PGF$_{1\alpha}$ or 2,3-dinor-6-oxo-PGF$_{1\alpha}$ are not representative of true prostacyclin synthesis in the organism. However, this possibility could only prove correct if the further metabolism of prostacyclin were determined by 15-hydroxydehydrogenase to a greater extent in the spontaneously hypertensive rats than in the Wistar rats. But this is not the case. In vitro studies have shown that the decisive enzyme, 15-hydroxydehydrogenase, is not increased

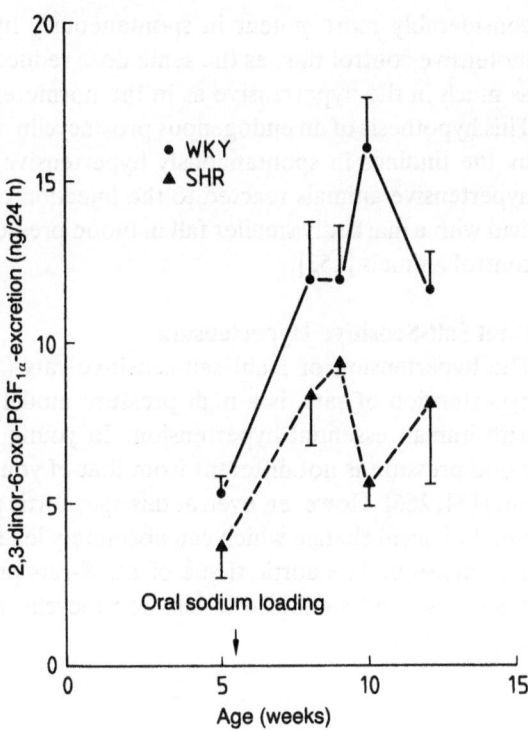

Fig. 29. Comparison of renal excretion of 2,3-dinor-6-oxo-PGF$_{1\alpha}$ in spontaneously hypertensive (*SHR*; ▲) and normotensive Wistar-Kyoto (*WKY*; ●) rats on normal diet and during oral sodium loading ($\bar{x} \pm$ SD) [158]

in activity in the spontaneously hypertensive rats, but rather exhibits a reduced activity in comparison with the Wistar rats [136, 201]. Therefore, an altered prostacyclin metabolism as the cause of the discrepancy between the in vitro and in vivo findings seems rather unlikely.

On the other hand, it is more probable that in the spontaneously hypertensive rats factors are lacking in the blood which normally stimulate vascular prostacyclin synthesis, or that their blood contains increased circulating factors which inhibit vascular prostacyclin synthesis in vivo. Such regulatory factors in the circulation have actually been demonstrated by various research teams [154, 207, 236]. These circulating factors elude in vitro studies and it is perfectly conceivable that because of this the results of the in vitro studies do not correspond to the in vivo situation of the organism and are to be interpreted with proper caution.

An argument for an endogenous deficiency of prostacyclin with an increased receptor sensitivity may be the finding that injected prostacyclin is

considerably more potent in spontaneously hypertensive rats than in normotensive control rats, as the same dose reduces the blood pressure by twice
as much in the hypertensive as in the normotensive animals (Fig. 30) [203].
This hypothesis of an endogenous prostacyclin deficiency is further supported
by the findings in spontaneously hypertensive rats, which showed that the
hypertensive animals reacted to the injection of a small dose of arachidonic
acid with a markedly smaller fall in blood pressure than did the normotensive
control animals [153].

Dahl Salt-Sensitive Hypertension

The hypertension of Dahl salt-sensitive rats (S-rats), like the spontaneous
hypertension of rats, is a high pressure model which at best is comparable
with human essential hypertension. In young S-rats on a low-salt diet the
blood pressure is not different from that of young R-rats (Dahl salt-resistant
rats) [64, 266]. However, even at this age, aortic prostaglandin synthesis shows
a pathological change which can absolutely lead to higher vascular tonus and
hypertension. The aortic tissue of the S-rats produces in vitro more thromboxane A_2 and significantly less prostacyclin than the tissue of the R-rats
(Fig. 31) [266].

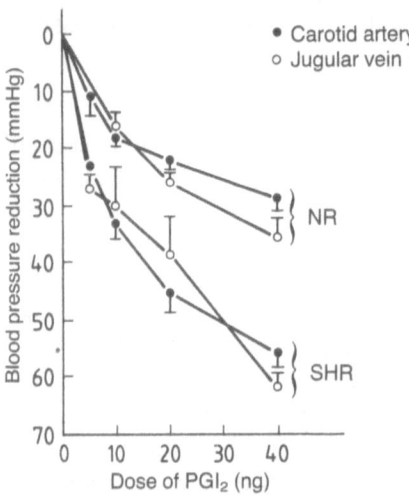

Fig. 30. Dose-effect relation between injected dose of prostacyclin and fall in blood
pressure in normotensive (*NR*, $n = 5$) and spontaneously hypertensive (*SHR*, $n = 5$)
rats. (•——•, injection into carotid artery; ○——○, injection into jugular vein;
$\bar{x} \pm$ SEM) [203]

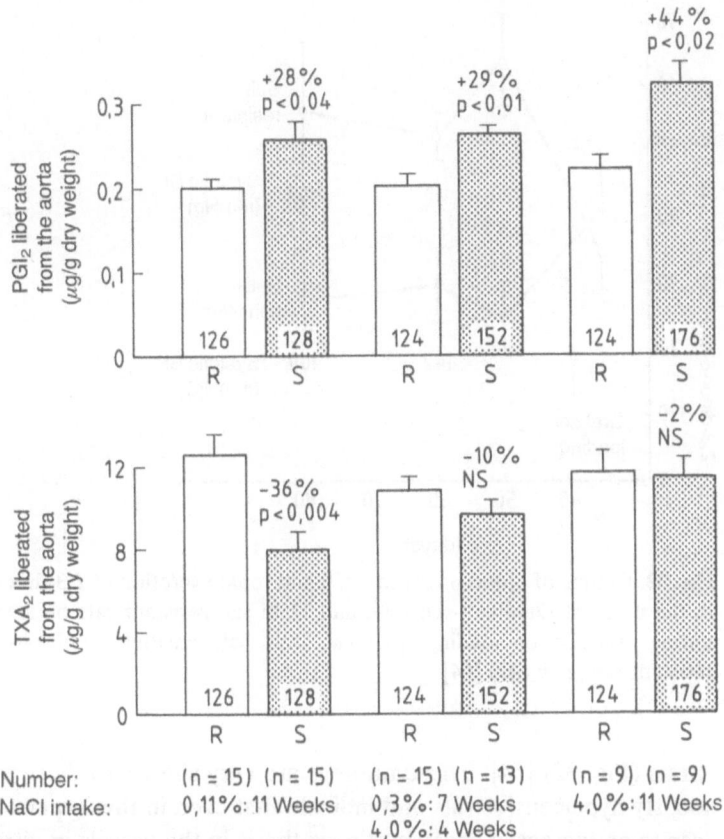

Number:	(n = 15) (n = 15)	(n = 15) (n = 13)	(n = 9) (n = 9)
NaCl intake:	0,11%: 11 Weeks	0,3%: 7 Weeks	4,0%: 11 Weeks
		4,0%: 4 Weeks	

Fig. 31. Comparison of aortic thromboxane A_2 and PGI_2 liberation in Dahl salt-resistant (*R*) and Dahl salt-sensitive (*S*) rats on different sodium intakes. The *numbers* in the *bars* give the mean blood pressure in the animals studied ($\bar{x} \pm$ SEM) [266]

However, at this stage there is still no difference in the renal excretion of prostacyclin metabolites in the two rat strains (Fig. 32) [64]. Dietetic sodium loading is known to provoke hypertension in the S-rats. With the development of hypertension aortic prostacyclin synthesis also markedly increases, and with markedly manifest hypertension it is ultimately equally expressed in both groups of animals. However, the synthesis of thromboxane A_2 also remains pathologically increased during sodium loading, so that the initial disproportion between thromboxane A_2 and prostacyclin in the aortic tissue continues to be demonstrable (Fig. 31) [266]. Under oral salt loading the renal excretion of prostacyclin metabolites does not increase, despite the increased aortic synthesis of prostacyclin, but even decreases as opposed to excretion in the

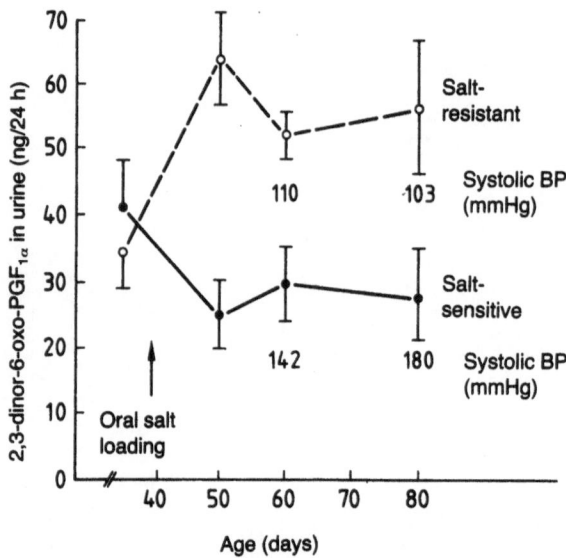

Fig. 32. Course of blood pressure (*BP*) and renal excretion of 2,3-dinor-6-oxo-PGE$_{1\alpha}$ in the urine of Dahl salt-sensitive and Dahl salt-resistant rats on standard diet and during oral sodium loading. (●——●, Dahl salt-sensitive rats; ○－－－○, Dahl salt-resistant rats; $\bar{x} \pm$ SD) [64]

R-rats (Fig. 32) [64]. These findings are very similar to those in the sponta-neously hypertensive rats and indicate that even in this hypertension model, despite an increased prostacyclin synthesis in the vessels in vitro, a systemic prostacyclin deficiency may develop in vivo. Consequently, the significance of this finding is to be assessed similarly as in the spontaneously hypertensive rats.

DOCA-Salt Hypertension

In DOCA-salt hypertension, it has been shown in studies in the rat that aortic prostacyclin synthesis is notably increased in vitro with the first manifestation of high blood pressure (Fig. 33) [75, 185]. However, after long-term duration of the hypertension the aortic synthesis of prostacyclin falls below the control value [185]. The initial increase in vascular prostacyclin formation with the development of hypertension is to be interpreted as a nonspecific reaction of the vessel wall to the increased pressure strain as the same type of reaction has been observed in other hypertension models. The secondary decrease in long-standing hypertension is very probably attributable to lesioning of the vascular system produced by the hypertension. On the basis of these not very

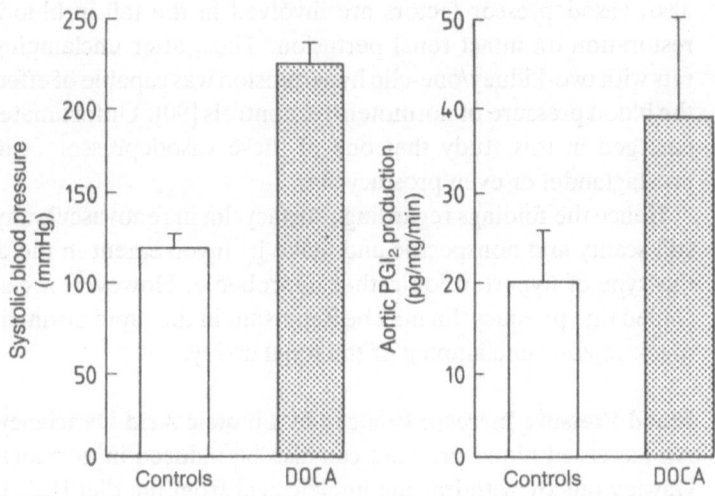

Fig. 33. Change of blood pressure and aortic prostacyclin production in DOCA-salt hypertension ($\bar{x} \pm$ SEM; $n = 9$) [75]

characteristic changes no specific significance for the pathogenesis of DOCA-salt hypertension can be attributed to prostacyclin.

Renovascular Hypertension

The available data about the significance of prostacyclin in renovascular hypertension is rather sparse. In the two-kidney/two-clip model of renovascular hypertension in the rat an increase in vascular prostacyclin synthesis with the development of the hypertension was initially observed [178]. However, in the course of the following 6 weeks vascular prostacyclin synthesis declined again though the blood pressure remained high. Also, in the one-kidney/one-clip model of renovascular hypertension and possibly also in the two-kidney/one-clip model, reduced phospholipase A_2 activity develops over time due to hitherto unknown factors, and this change may lead to a deficiency of vascular prostacyclin [165]. Less speculative are the findings after unclamping of the renal artery in the one-kidney/one-clip model. Here a rapid increase in the activity of phospholipase A_2 with a subsequent increase in vascular prostacyclin synthesis can regularly be demonstrated [165, 268, 269]. Pretreatment of the animals with indomethacin markedly delays the fall in blood pressure after unclamping in this hypertension model [268]. In the two-kidney/one-clip model of renovascular hypertension no direct evidence has yet been found of prostacyclin involvement in the renormalization of blood pressure after unclamping. However, there is evidence that, in this hypertension model

45

also, vasodepressor factors are involved in the fall in blood pressure after restoration on intact renal perfusion. Thus, after unclamping, the blood of rats with two-kidney/one-clip hypertension was capable of effectively reducing the blood pressure of normotensive controls [90]. Unfortunately, no evidence emerged in this study that one of these vasodepressor factors might be a prostaglandin or even prostacyclin.

Hence the findings regarding prostacyclin in renovascular hypertension are still scanty and nonspecific and make its involvement in the development of this type of hypertension rather improbable. However, it cannot yet be excluded that prostacyclin may be important in the rapid normalization of blood pressure after unclamping of the renal artery.

Blood Pressure Increase Induced by Linoleic Acid Deficiency

An increased blood pressure can also be induced in normotensive Sprague-Dawley rats by withdrawing linoleic acid from the diet [52]. In these studies a continuous and statistically significant increase in systolic blood pressure

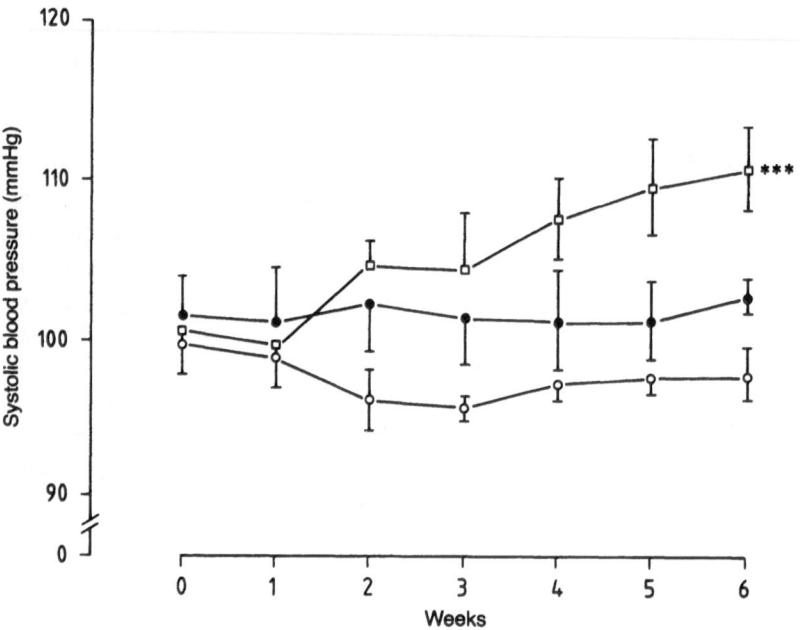

Fig. 34. Behaviour of systolic blood pressure in Sprague-Dawley rats with alteration of dietetic intake of linoleic acid. The blood pressure rose markedly with linoleic acid deprivation (□), remained unchanged with 5% of energy intake coming from linoleic acid (●) and fell slightly but not significantly with 9 energy per cent linoleic acid in the diet (○). ($\bar{x} \pm$ SEM; *** $P < 0.005$ compared with diet containing linoleic acid) [52]

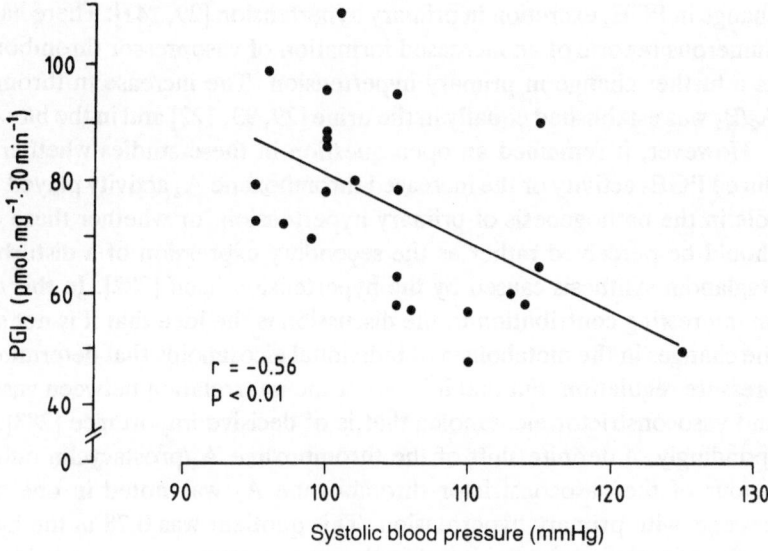

Fig. 35. Correlation between increase in blood pressure and decline in prostacyclin synthesis in isolated aortic tissue evoked by variations in dietetic linoleic acid intake after 6 weeks [52]

developed after 6 weeks of linoleic acid deprivation (Fig. 34). This increase was associated with a simultaneous increase in thrombocytic thromboxane synthesis and a decline in aortic prostacyclin synthesis, a decline which was closely correlated ($P < 0.01$) in these experiments with the increase in the animals' systolic blood pressure (Fig. 35). In this model of systolic blood pressure increase there was no question of any other hypertensive mechanism, so that these findings provided the first valuable evidence that the eicosanoids, among them particularly vascular prostacyclin, may be involved in regulation of the systemic blood pressure.

4.2 Arterial Hypertension

Primary Hypertension

Numerous investigations have been made to study the changes in the prostaglandins in essential or primary human hypertension. These were generally at one in finding an obvious reduction of renal PGE_2 excretion [234, 257, 281, 282] shown to be correlated with the degree of severity of the hypertension [283]. The findings were rather more marked in the so-called "low renin" type of hypertension [3, 29, 78, 257]. Only a few studies found no significant change in PGE_2 excretion in primary hypertension [29, 141]. There have been numerous reports of an increased formation of vasopressor thromboxane A_2 as a further change in primary hypertension. The increase in thromboxane A_2/B_2 was established equally in the urine [29, 93, 122] and in the blood [122].

However, it remained an open question in these studies whether the reduced PGE_2 activity or the increased thromboxane A_2 activity played a causal role in the pathogenesis of primary hypertension, or whether these changes should be perceived rather as the secondary expression of a disturbed prostaglandin synthesis caused by the hypertension itself [282]. In this context, an interesting contribution to the discussion is the idea that it is not so much the changes in the metabolism of individual eicosanoids that determine blood pressure regulation, but that it is rather the interrelation between vasodilator and vasoconstrictor eicosanoids that is of decisive importance [283]. Correspondingly, a definite shift of the thromboxane A_2/prostacyclin quotient in favour of the vasoconstrictor thromboxane A_2 was noted in one study of patients with primary hypertension. This quotient was 0.78 in the hypertensives, more than twice as high as in the normotensive control individuals with a quotient of only 0.29 [93]. A similarly marked shift of this quotient was also found in a study of respiratory insufficiency in the newborn with hypertension during extracorporeal circulation [237]. In these patients, during extracorporeal oxygenation of the blood, there developed a marked increase in thromboxane by about 50% and a dramatic fall in the blood prostacyclin to 20% of the initial value.

Unfortunately, no further studies are presently available with simultaneous determination of thromboxane A_2/B_2 and prostacyclin in patients with primary hypertension. In the other studies concerned with the behaviour of prostacyclin in primary hypertension, only this one eicosanoid was determined through its metabolite 6-oxo-$PGF_{1\alpha}$. In an earlier study of a small series of patients, a significantly lower excretion of prostacyclin in the urine was found in hypertensive than in normotensive individuals [92]. In a larger series studied by the same author the differential trend was still present, but without statistical significance [93]. Variable changes in prostacyclin concentration in the blood of patients with primary hypertension have been observed. Thus, one group reported markedly elevated prostacyclin concentrations [254], another found unchanged levels with a normal response to bendroflumethiazide [75, 114] and two other teams found a markedly lowered prostacyclin concentration in the blood [237, 265].

All the studies took as control groups of normotensive subjects of comparable age and sex. In recent studies there was a significant inverse correlation between the concentration of the prostacyclin metabolite 6-oxo-$PGF_{1\alpha}$ and the blood pressure (Fig. 34), but not with plasma renin activity [265]. However, in a recently completed study the reduction of renal prostacyclin excretion in essential hypertension was confirmed by the most modern measurement techniques [127]. This finding persisted even when the reduced excretion of prostacyclin metabolites was calculated in terms of creatinine excretion (Fig. 36). It is a particularly interesting observation that the urinary excretion of prostacyclin metabolites had a strictly linear correlation with the mean arterial pressure of the patients (Fig. 37). The interpretation of these findings about prostacyclin in primary hypertension is problematic as it is not certain that the circulating or renally excreted amounts of prostacyclin represent the local rate of synthesis in the vessels [33]. Thus a disturbed prostacyclin metabolism in hypertension, as has been described for the reduced activity of 15-hydroxy-dehydrogenase [136, 201], might produce normal or even elevated plasma concentrations despite reduced prostacyclin synthesis and thereby falsely simulate unimpaired prostacyclin formation. Also, an alteration of vascular prostacyclin secretion rate could result in normal circulating levels although lower biological activity may exist in the tissues themselves. For these reasons, it seems indispensable in connexion with the vascular prostaglandin, the prostacyclin, to establish its synthesis, secretion and metabolism

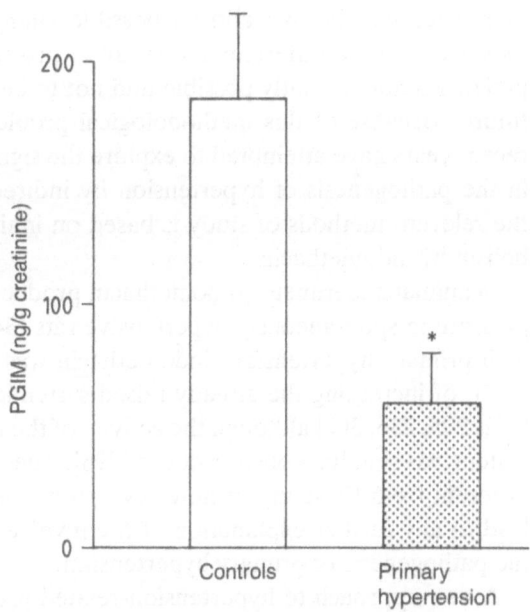

Fig. 36. Comparison of renal excretion of prostacyclin metabolites (*PGIM*) in the urine of control individuals and patients with mild primary hypertension ($\bar{x} \pm$ SEM; * $P < 0.05$) [12]

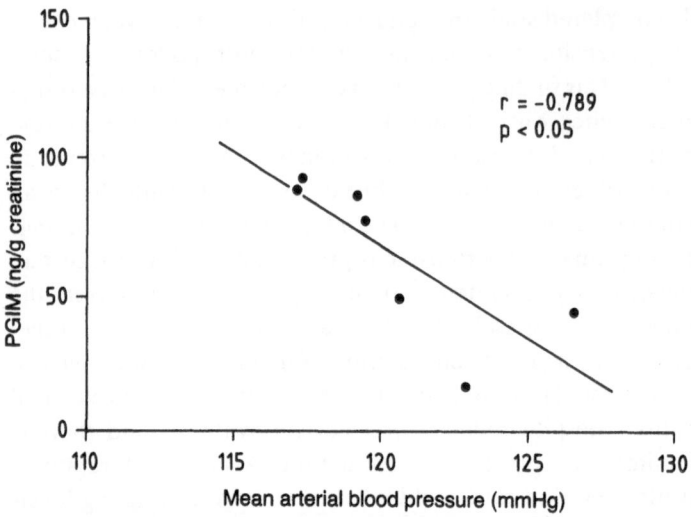

Fig. 37. Correlation of mean arterial blood pressure and renal excretion of prostacyclin metabolites (*PGIM*) in the urine of patients with primary hypertension [12]

in order finally to arrive at a comprehensive thesis as to the biological activity of prostacyclin in vivo and its possible changes in primary hypertension. However, such a differentiated study of prostacyclin metabolism in vivo in patients is not currently possible und not to be conducted in the foreseeable future. Because of this methodological problem numerous investigators in recent years have attempted to explore the significance of the prostaglandins in the pathogenesis of hypertension by indirect means. The commonest of the relevant methods of study is based on inhibition of prostaglandin metabolism by indomethacin.

In animal experiments indomethacin produces a marked increase in blood pressure in spontaneously hypertensive rats [34, 146, 214]. Also, in patients with primary hypertension, indomethacin was capable, with few exceptions [227], of increasing the already raised systemic blood pressure even further [151, 205, 236, 300] although the activity of the renin-angiotensin-aldosterone system was simultaneously reduced [296]. These findings were not noticeably different from those in normotensive probands [290] and did not ultimately lead to any further explanation of the involvement of the prostaglandins in the pathogenesis of primary hypertension.

A new approach to hypertension-related prostaglandin research was provided by the demonstration of prostacyclin in brain tissue, the choroid plexus and the cerebrospinal fluid [86]. According to these studies the prostacyclin concentration in the CSF is even many times greater than in the blood.

Prostacyclin also seems to antagonize the renin-angiotensin system in the cerebral tissue, for inhibition of its synthesis by indomethacin leads promptly to an increased blood pressure reaction to renin injected into the cerebral ventricles [232]. This central action of prostacyclin might under certain circumstances be of great importance in the regulation of systemic blood pressure as a local cerebral deficiency of prostacyclin would abolish its physiological antagonism to the action of cerebral angiotensin II. Under these conditions angiotensin II could have an increased effect in raising blood pressure and evoking a centrally induced hypertension. But this interesting hypothesis, too, calls for further experimental confirmation.

Pregnancy-Associated Hypertension
In pregnancy hypertension can become manifest for the first time or a preexisting hypertension may deteriorate. The mechanism underlying pregnancy hypertension is still unknown and is very probably multifactorial. Normally in pregnancy the responsiveness of the vessels to angiotensin II is decreased, possibly as the result of increased vascular prostacyclin synthesis [67, 228]. An increased sensitivity of the vessels to angiotensin II has proved to be a predictive factor for the early recognition of pregnancy-associated hypertension as it is usually demonstrable before hypertension becomes evident [81]. However, this test is not clinically applicable because of possible risk to the fetus. The increased responsiveness of the vessels to angiotensin II may be based entirely on reduced prostacyclin counter-regulation, for in women who develop hypertension during their pregnancy the renal excretion of prostacyclin metabolites is markedly less than in healthy pregnant women (Fig. 38) [180]. The changes in prostacyclin levels run parallel with the increased sensitivity of the vessels to angiotensin II even before hypertension becomes evident. Hence, serial observations of prostacyclin metabolism may be clinically useful and provide an early indication of developing hypertension. Pharmacological stimulation of prostacyclin synthesis, as by the inhibition of thromboxane synthetase by low doses of acetylsalicylic acid (80 mg), enhances the counter-regulatory potency of prostacyclin against angiotensin II and markedly reduces the vascular sensitivity to this peptide [228]. The favourable effect of acetylsalicylic acid on pregnancy hypertension can be accounted for by the inhibition of thromboxane A_2 and the reinforcement of prostacyclin [277, 278]. The question as to whether this therapeutical all effect can also be attributed to prostacyclin and other prostacyclin-stimulating substances remains open at the present time as further studies are still lacking.

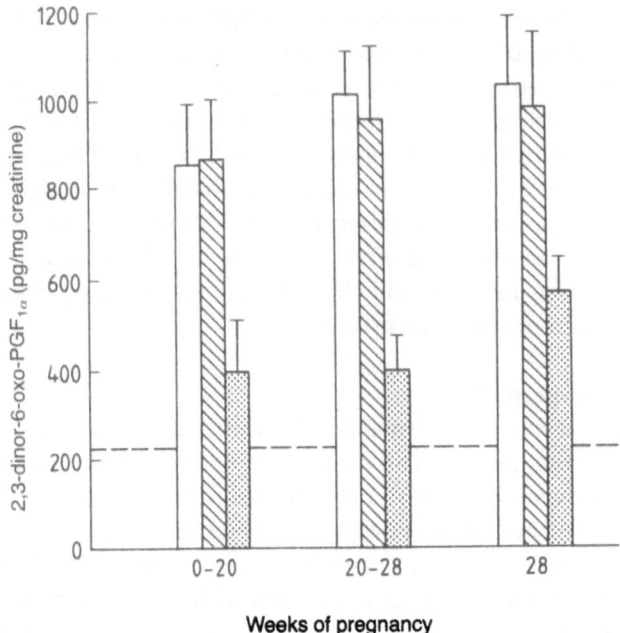

Fig. 38. Renal excretion of 2,3-dinor-6-oxo-PGF$_{1\alpha}$ during pregnancy in normotensive women (*open bars*; $n = 22$), patients with exercise hypertension (*hatched bars*; $n = 22$) and women with pregnancy-induced hypertension (*stippled bars*; $n = 12$). The *interrupted transverse line* shows the 95% confidence limit for normal, age-paired, non-pregnant controls ($\bar{x} \pm$ SEM) [67]

Interrelation Between Hypertension and Atherosclerosis

Generalized atherosclerosis is the commonest vascular complication of arterial hypertension and, conversely, a preexisting atherosclerosis can be complicated by the development of hypertension. Prostacyclin may be of very considerable importance in this interrelation since it can no longer be synthesized in normal concentrations by vessels affected by atherosclerosis [47, 95, 138, 139]. In one study the formation of prostacyclin in the vessels was reduced by over 50% [47]. However, thromboxane synthesis in the platelets and other tissues remains unimpaired [95]. In this manner vascular atherosclerosis leads to a disequilibrium between normal thrombocytic thromboxane A$_2$ and reduced vascular prostacyclin. The consequence of this change is, inter alia, an increased deposition of cholesterol esters in the vessel wall and an enhanced adhesion of platelets to the damaged endothelium. Thereby the platelets can liberate increased mitogenic factors locally which stimulate proliferation of the vascular smooth muscle and hence further increase the development of atherosclerotic plaques [133]. As regards the hypertension, it may be postulated that because of the disequilibrium between vascular prostacyclin and thrombocytic thromboxane A_2 the tonus of the affected vessels is also subject to an increase. By means of this mechanism atherosclerosis could serve to precipitate hypertension or to enhance and further promote a preexisting hypertension. These hypotheses may possibly have important clinical implications related to substitution treatment with prostacyclin in hypertension and atherosclerosis. Pharmacological studies have already shown the positive effect of prostacyclin on atherosclerosis (in vitro) and on blood pressure (in vivo) [193, 231], but unfortunately adequate long-term studies on this problem are still not available.

4.3 Influence of Antihypertensive Agents

Since prostacyclin is the most potent vasodilator among the prostaglandins and also constitutes the main prostaglandin of the vessels, the treatment of hypertension in the past has not failed to conceive that stimulation of prostacyclin might lead to blood pressure reduction or at least reinforce other blood pressure-reducing mechanisms. Such considerations referred particularly to antihypertensive agents such as diuretics, unsaturated fatty acid diets and inhibitors of angiotensin I converting enzyme.

Diets
As regards diets with polyunsaturated vegetable fatty acids or omega-3-fatty acids (eicosapentaenoic acid), it has been shown that these stimulate the synthesis of PGI_2 (prostacyclin) or PGI_3 and act to reduce blood pressure (see Chap. 2.3). Accordingly, in patients with primary hypertension a marked reduction of blood pressure (over 10% of the initial value) was obtained with a diet containing polyunsaturated vegetable fatty acids [41, 216] or omega-3-fatty acids (eicosapentaenoic acids) [190, 243]. The responsiveness of the vessels to pressor hormones was also reduced by unsaturated fatty acid diets [152, 233]. In addition to these favourable effects on the blood pressure and its regulation, it was established that a further advantage of these diets was a decline in the serum cholesterol. The HDL fraction of the cholesterol fell slightly or remained unaltered, while the LDL fraction fell drastically [57].

Diuretics
The significance of prostaglandins in the blood pressure-reducing and diuretic action of diuretics has usually been studied indirectly by inhibition of prostaglandin synthesis with indomethacin. These studies showed that following

indomethacin there was a weakening of the action of furosemide, triamterene, acetazolamide and, to a lesser extent, hydrochlorothiazide [65, 151, 205, 279]. However, these studies leave it unsettled whether indomethacin reduces the action of diuretics only by inhibiting prostaglandin synthesis or whether it can itself induce sodium retention. The latter could be responsible for a reduction of diuretic action by means of a physiological antagonism, quite independently of the prostaglandin system. The same studies showed that prostaglandin inhibition had no effect on the diuretic action of amiloride and spironolactone. Direct measurements of prostaglandins in the blood and urine after diuretic administration showed a stimulation of PGE_2 synthesis for triamterene, furosemide, hydrochlorothiazide and indapamide, whereas no such stimulation was demonstrable for amiloride [66, 142, 229, 251].

The data concerning prostacyclin is sparse. Thus an increased prostacyclin activity has been demonstrated in both the plasma (Fig. 39) and the urine after bendroflumethiazide therapy [284]. In vitro, furosemide stimulates pro-

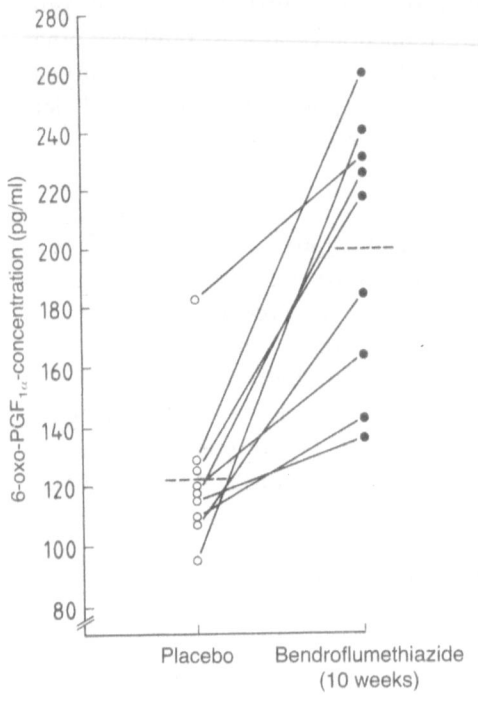

Fig. 39. Plasma levels of 6-oxo-PGF$_{1\alpha}$ after placebo and 10 weeks' treatment with 10 mg bendroflumethiazide daily in nine hypertensive patients. The *interrupted transverse lines* represent the mean values [284]

stacyclin synthesis in aortic tissue [53, 252] and in the microsomes of the seminal vesicles of sheep [83]. No significant stimulation of aortic prostacyclin synthesis in vitro could be shown for muzolimine, piretanide and bemetizide [53]. However, on closer consideration it remains very doubtful whether the diuretic-induced stimulation of prostaglandins is physiologically important as it is regularly associated with a significantly more marked stimulation of the vasoconstrictor hormonal system, especially the renin-angiotensin system and the mineralocorticoids.

Beta-Blockers

The action of beta-receptor antagonists on vascular prostacyclin synthesis has not been much investigated. Up to now, only two studies [12, 73] have reported a direct stimulation of prostacyclin by beta-receptor blockade with propranolol. In a further study, after pretreatment with mepindolol [131], it was observed that prostacyclin synthesis was more markedly stimulated by arachidonic acid after blockade of the beta-receptors than with intact unin-hibited receptors. In further studies with inhibition of prostaglandin synthesis by indomethacin, a considerable diminution of the blood pressure-reducing action of propranolol was noted [12, 55, 151, 279]. However, these findings can only be regarded as indirect evidence of a global involvement of prosta-glandins in the reduction of blood pressure by beta-blockers, especially as it cannot be excluded that indomethacin produces this weakening of the action of beta-receptor blockers only via its own blood pressure-enhancing proper-ties [205] and not by directly interfering with the mechanism of action of these agents.

Calcium Antagonists

The calcium antagonists develop in vitro and in vivo numerous properties which are very similar to the physiological effects of prostacyclin. These include an antiaggregatory action on the platelets, inhibition of thrombocytic thromboxane synthesis, inhibition of cholesterol storage in the macrophages, as well as potent vasodilatation and blood pressure reduction [140]. The available reports show that these effects, though with variable trends, are equally valid for all calcium antagonists, but are particularly uniform and clearly demonstrable for calcium antagonists of the nifedipine type. Consis-tent with the results of these studies is the fact that calcium antagonists can also be shown to stimulate vascular prostacyclin synthesis, a stimulation observed both in vitro [124, 166] and in vivo [91]. In a platelet/arterial model, vascular prostacyclin stimulation by calcium antagonists was even associated with an inhibition of thrombocytic thromboxane formation [118, 249]. How-ever, unlike prostacyclin, calcium antagonists exert their prostacyclin-like effects without stimulation of intracellular cAMP [140]. This finding argues for a direct prostacyclinlike action of the calcium antagonists themselves and legitimately raises the question whether the observed stimulation of vascular prostacyclin synthesis by calcium antagonists can really be of additional clinical relevance.

Angiotensin I Converting Enzyme Inhibitors

The angiotensin I converting enzyme (ACE) forms the biologically active angiotensin II from angiotensin I. It simultaneously inactivates the kinins by splitting off a dipeptide. Inhibition of this enzyme leads subsequently to a decline in angiotensin II concentration and kinin accumulation. Inhibitors of ACE can reduce the blood pressure by both these mechanisms. The blood pressure-reducing action of the kinins is possibly reinforced by a stimulation of prostaglandin synthesis since bradykinin can stimulate phospholipase A_2 (Fig. 40). Corresponding to this mode of action of bradykinin, a markedly

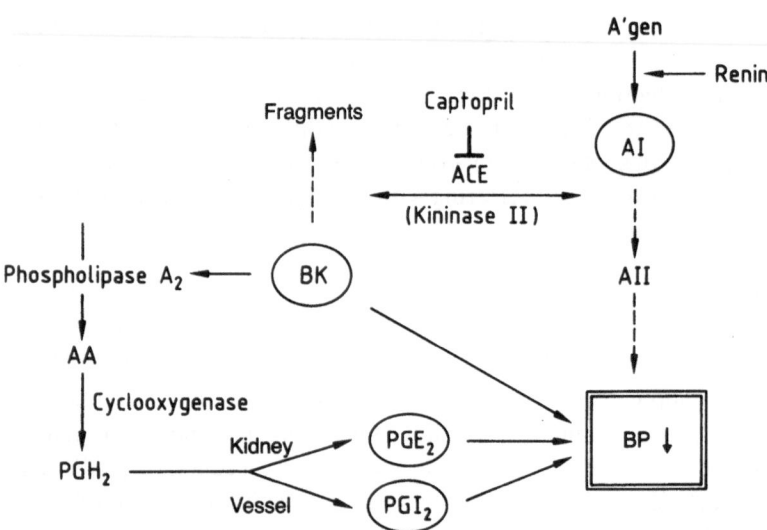

Fig. 40. Interrelation between the renin-angiotensin system, bradykinin and prostaglandins. The ACE inhibitor captopril inhibits the renin-angiotensin system and stops the conversion of angiotensin I (*AI*). Captopril further prevents the breakdown of kinins and thus leads to an accumulation of bradykinin (*BK*). In turn, the reinforced action of bradykinin now stimulates the synthesis of prostaglandins PGE_2 and PGI_2. All three effects (inhibition of the renin-angiotensin system, potentiation of kinins and stimulation of prostaglandins) work compatibly and produce a fall in systemic blood pressure (*BP*)

Table 4. Influence of captopril on basal and bradykinin-stimulated liberation of arachidonic acid and PGE$_2$ synthesis in cell cultures of renal medullary interstitial tissue. ($\bar{x} \pm$ SEM)

Protocol	n	Arachidonic acid formation (fmol/μg protein/h)	PGE$_2$ synthesis (ng/μg protein/h)
Control	8	42 ± 4	0,3 ± 0,1
Captopril (7,5 μM)	8	3425 ± 269**	2,4 ± 0,4**
Bradykinin (20 nM)	8	3428 ± 427**	3,0 ± 0,6**
Captopril + Bradykinin	8	21629 ± 668**	8,1 ± 0,8**

** $P < 0.01$

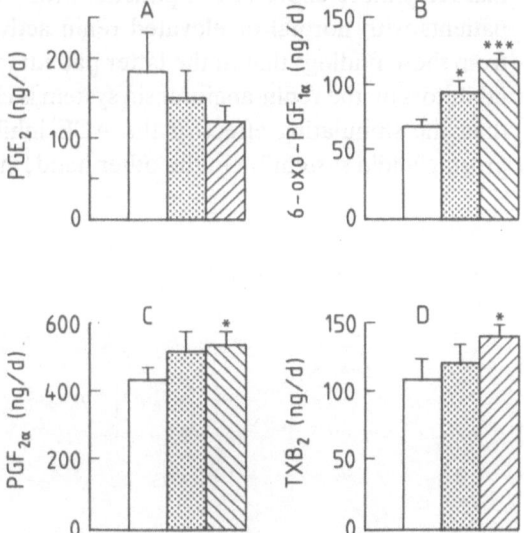

Fig. 41. Excretion of PGE$_2$ **(A)**, 6-oxo-PGF$_{1\alpha}$ **(B)**, PGF$_{2\alpha}$ **(C)** and TXB$_2$ **(D)** in the 24-h urine in spontaneously hypertensive rats at the 5th–6th day of captopril treatment. *Open bars,* control group; *stippled bars,* captopril 20 mg/kg; *hatched bars,* captopril 100 mg/kg ($\bar{x} \pm$ SEM; * $P < 0.05$; *** $P < 0.001$) [224]

increased cellular liberation of arachidonic acid can be observed after the administration of ACE inhibitors (Table 4) [303]. Hence an increased synthesis of PGE$_2$ occurs in the interstitial and tubular renal tissue [3, 177, 255, 274, 304], whereas a stimulation of vascular prostacyclin is noted in the vessels of the systemic circulation and the renal glomeruli [80, 188, 224, 225, 304]. These findings apply to all ACE inhibitors, such as teprotide, captopril and enalapril.

Unequivocal stimulation of both eicosanoids has been found in only a few studies [224, 255, 276]. However, lowered PGE_2 values are not absolute evidence of deficient stimulation of PGE_2 as the lower values may result from a change in PGE_2 metabolism. Bradykinin also activates 9-keto-reductase and thus promotes the conversion of PGE_2 into $PGF_{2\alpha}$, as was clear from one of the studies on spontaneously hypertensive rats (Fig. 41) [224].

The importance of the prostaglandins and particularly of vascular prostacyclin in the blood pressure-reducing action of the ACE inhibitors is especially demonstrated when these agents are administered simultaneously with indomethacin. After the inhibition of prostaglandin synthesis the blood pressure fall is usually diminished by the ACE inhibitors (Fig. 42). This finding applies to normotensive and hypertensive individuals [3, 88, 192, 241, 297] and is markedly more expressed in patients with "low renin" hypertension than in patients with normal or elevated renin activity [3, 88]. It may be deduced from these findings that in the latter patients the inhibitory effect of the ACE inhibitors on the renin-angiotensin system is clearly expressed more markedly than the stimulating effect of the ACE inhibitors on the "kallikrein-kinin-prostaglandin system". On the other hand, in patients with lower basal renin

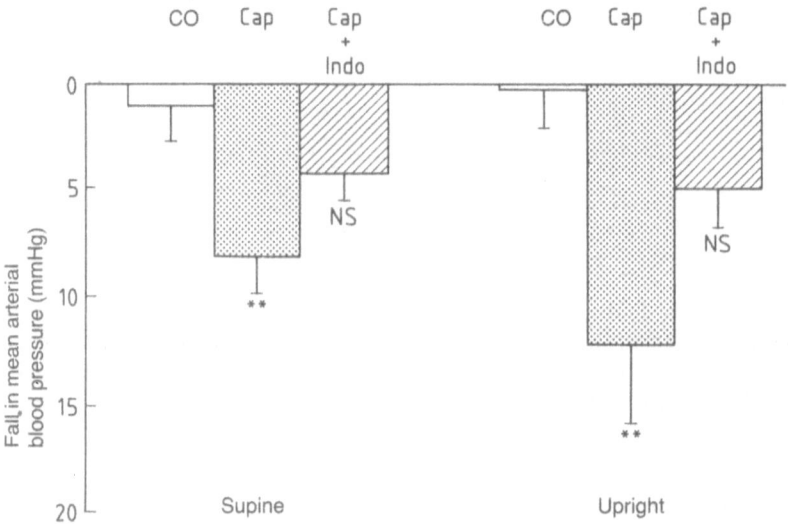

Fig. 42. Comparison of reactions of arterial blood pressure to captopril (*Cap;* 25 mg orally) in nine healthy subjects lying *(left)* and standing *(right)*. Pretreatment with indomethacin *(Indo)* markedly reduces the fall in blood pressure produced by captopril, so that it is no longer significantly *(NS)* different from that of the placebo control group *(CO)*; ($\bar{x} \pm$ SEM; ** $P < 0.01$ vs control group) [241]

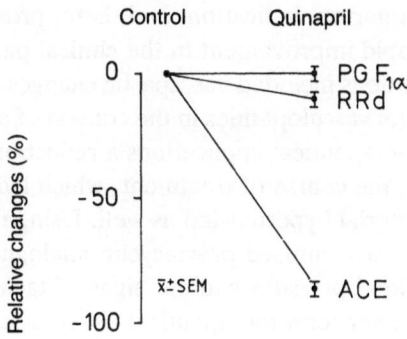

Fig. 43. Influence of 12 weeks' treatment with quinapril on the activity of the angiotensin-converting enzyme *(ACE)*, the diastolic blood pressure *(RRd)* and the concentration of the prostacyclin metabolite 6-oxo-PGF$_{1\alpha}$ (PGF$_{1\alpha}$) in the urine of patients with essential hypertension [226]

activity the conditions are quite reversed, and in this group the stimulating effect of the ACE inhibitors on the kinins and prostaglandins, especially vascular-formed prostacyclin, may share the responsibility for the blood pressure-reducing properties of this group of substances.

Unfortunately, however, the results of all these studies must be interpreted with the greatest caution because of the specific blood pressure-raising effect of indomethacin. It adds to the difficulty that it has not yet been possible to demonstrate persistent long-term kinin stimulation by ACE inhibitors. Although the fall in blood pressure produced by captopril in the short term was diminished by pretreatment of the patients with aprotinin, a potent kallikrein inhibitor, after 4 weeks of captopril treatment aprotinin had had no effect at all on the blood pressure of the treated patients [200]. Even the prostacyclin stimulation often described in short-term experiments was no longer demonstrable after a longer period of treatment (quinapril for 12 weeks) (Fig. 43) although the inhibition of ACE activity and the fall in blood pressure remained undiminished [226]. These first results of long-term studies seriously call in question a long-term stimulation of the kinins and hence also of prostacyclins by ACE inhibitors and suggest that in the long-term use of these substances the inhibition of the renin-angiotensin system comes to occupy the foreground of the blood pressure influence of these substances.

4.4 Employment of Prostacyclin, Prostacyclin Analogues and Prostacyclin-Stimulating Substances in Hypertension

Prostacyclin and Prostacyclin Analogues

The therapeutic employment of prostacyclin or its analogues began quite soon after their discovery. Occlusive arterial disease soon emerged as the most important indication, and, here, prostacyclin and its derivatives often led to rapid improvement in the clinical picture [45, 244, 256]. Other clinical indications included vasospastic changes as in Raynaud's syndrome or in peripheral vasculopathies in the context of a systemic collagenosis [215]. With these therapeutical applications a reduction of blood pressure also often occurred in the course of treatment, which led to the employment of prostacyclin for arterial hypertension as well. Using the model of experimental hypertension in rats, infused prostacyclin analogue iloprost produced a long-term fall in blood pressure without signs of tachyphylaxis (Fig. 44) [231]. However, its longer term therapeutical use in arterial hypertension was hampered by the exclusively parenteral mode of administration of prostacyclin and its analogues and by the regular appearance of undesirable side effects with higher doses (8 ng/kg per min or more) [179]. These problems have not yet been satisfactorily resolved for prostacyclin and all its derivatives, so that the routine clinical treatment of hypertension with this group of substances is still excluded at present.

Prostacyclin-Stimulating Substances

Not only does prostacyclin reduce blood pressure in patients with hypertension, moreover, its broad action profile also confers on it further favourable

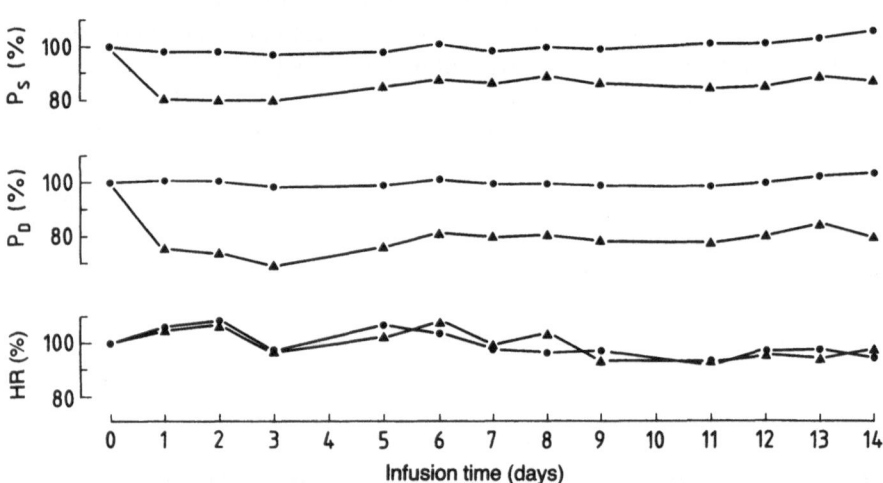

Fig. 44. Persistent reduction of systolic (P_S) and diastolic (P_D) blood pressure in spontaneously hypertensive rats ($n = 5$) during a 14-day infusion of the prostacyclin analogue iloprost (10 µg/min). The heart rate *(HR)* shows no significant changes. (•——•, solvent group; ▲——▲, iloprost group; mean values) [231]

properties which enable it to reduce other cardiovascular risks in these patients as well. These include the reduction of the sensitivity of the vessels to vasopressor agents, the cytoprotective action on the heart, the reduction in platelet aggregation and adhesion, as well as the property of counteracting the progress of atherosclerosis by changes in cholesterol metabolism in the vascular musculature (see Chap. 3). Since prostacyclin itself had proved unsuitable for antihypertensive therapy, interest was turned to a search for substances capable of specifically stimulating vascular prostacyclin.

Primary consideration in these studies was given to the older findings relating to the diuretics or ACE inhibitors, as these lead more frequently than any other group of agents to stimulation of prostacyclin synthesis. However, the problems previously described in connexion with these drugs make their use unsuitable for the deliberate stimulation of prostacyclin synthesis and initiated intensive research in this field. A new substance has now been successfully developed which produces stimulation of prostacyclin synthesis in vivo persisting for several hours (Fig. 46). This substance is cicletanine, a furopyridine derivative (Fig. 45). Cicletanine stimulates vascular prostacyclin synthesis in vitro and in vivo [50, 98] and can thus produce a marked vasodilatation [24]. Its main mechanism of action appears as an increased activity

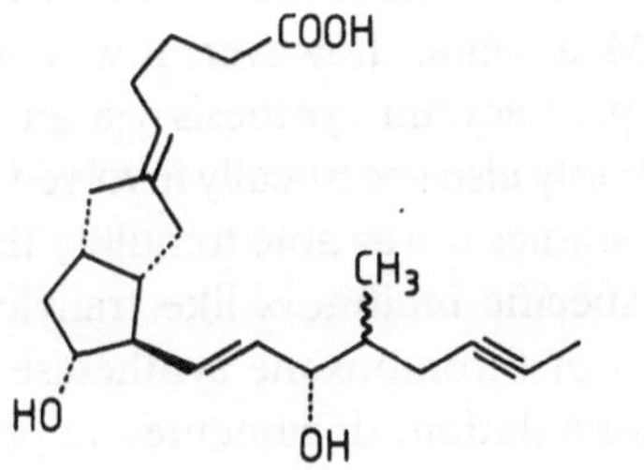

Iloprost

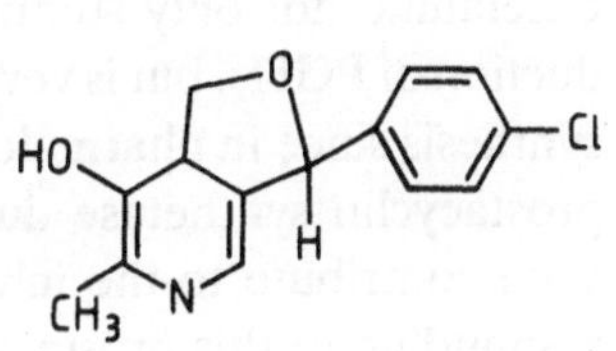

Cicletanine

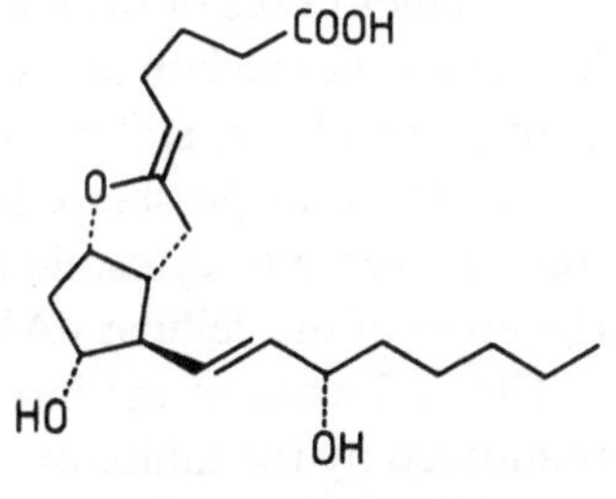

Fig. 45. Structural formulae of therapeutically applicable prostacyclin derivatives such as iloprost, epoprostenol (*PGI₂*), and the prostacyclin-stimulating substance cicletanine

Epoprostenol (PGI₂)

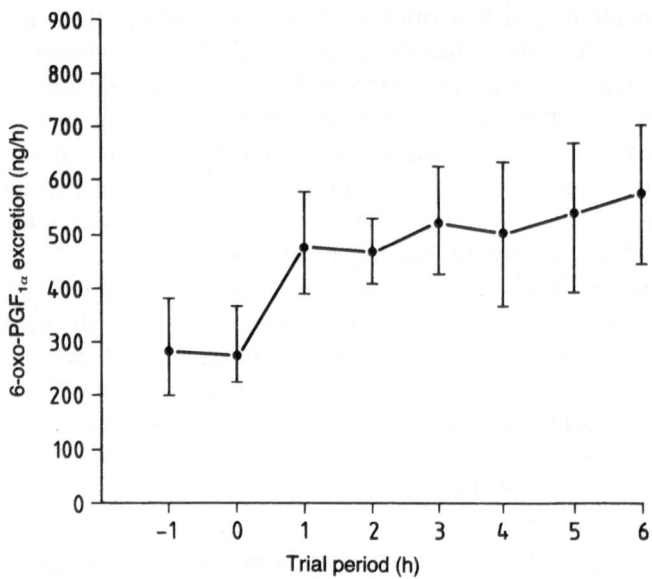

Fig. 46. Persistent increase in renal prostacyclin excretion in healthy subjects after 150 mg cicletanine orally ($\bar{x} \pm$ SD) [98]

of the arachidonic acid cascade with increased liberation of cyclooxygenase products [37, 50, 82, 98, 128]. Meanwhile, however, it was also shown that cicletanine not only stimulates prostacyclin synthesis via an increased production of PGH_2, but is very probably also specifically involved in prostacyclin synthesis since in pharmalogical studies it was able to nullify the inhibition of prostacyclin synthetase due to specific inhibitors like tranylcypromine and even contribute to the inhibition of thromboxane synthetase [21, 23]. Corresponding to this prostacyclin stimulation, documented in pharmacological studies, other prostacyclin effects could also be induced by cicletanine: a reduced responsiveness of the vessels to vasopressor substances and myocardial cytoprotection in acute ischaemia [51, 123, 128, 143].

In higher doses of over 100 mg, cicletanine also produces a fall in the free intracytosolic calcium of the vascular muscle cells, the underlying mechanism of this effect being still unclear. However, it could be regarded as the natural consequence of prostacyclin stimulation [30, 82, 89] since prostacyclin can transfer free intracytosolic calcium into the calcium store of the cell via an elevation of the cellular cAMP content [140, 302].

This influence of the intracytosolic calcium of the vascular muscle cells is reinforced by the inhibitory action of cicletanine on the H_1-receptors, as has been shown in a number of pharmacological studies [149, 156, 230]. A central inhibitory effect of cicletanine on the H_1 receptors has not yet been demonstrated [209]. A further observed effect of cicletanine was an increase of diuresis and natriuresis. This effect was demonstrated only for higher doses (100 mg and over) and was usually accompanied by a marked stimulation of renal prostacyclin synthesis [98, 99]. Low doses of cicletanine (50 mg) still showed a definite blood pressure-reducing action, but without demonstrable diurectic effect (Fig. 47). Thus, it was established in spontaneously hypertensive rats that cicletanine initially in low doses of 0.1–3.0 mg/kg only produced a fall in blood presure, and that it was only in higher doses of 10–30 mg/kg that it additionally exerted diuretic action (Fig. 48) [30].

All the described effects – vasodilatation, reduction of intracytosolic calcium and stimulation of diuresis and natriuresis – might ultimately be attributable to a single mechanism of action, i.e. stimulation of prostacyclin synthesis, though this remains to be placed in context in future pharmacological studies. Interpreted in this sense, all these effects taken together produce a powerful reduction of blood pressure, as has also been repeatedly described in spontaneously hypertensive rats or patients with essential hypertension [17, 20, 24, 25]. The blood pressure reduction with cicletanine in low dosage of

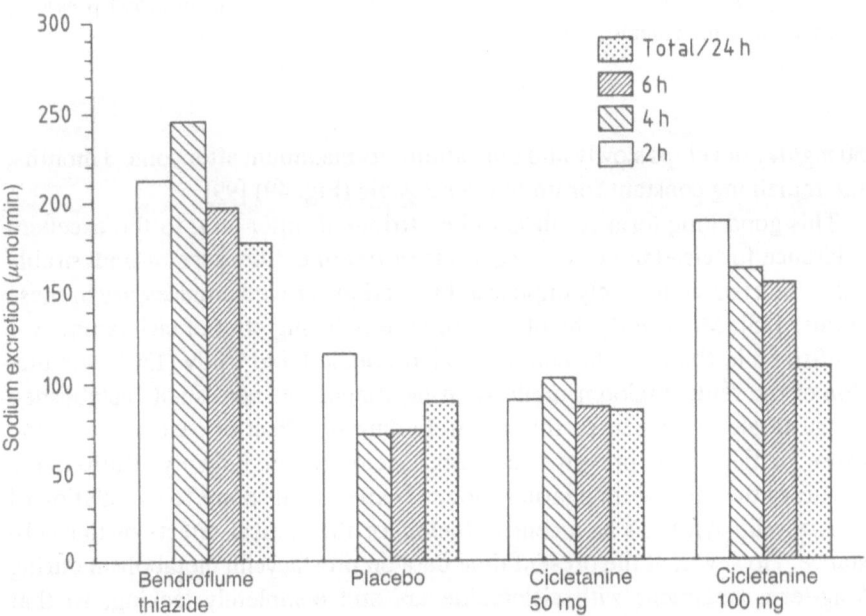

Fig. 47. Mean urinary sodium excretion in patients with mild hypertension after a single dose of 50 or 100 mg cicletanine, 5 mg bendroflumethiazide or placebo [99]

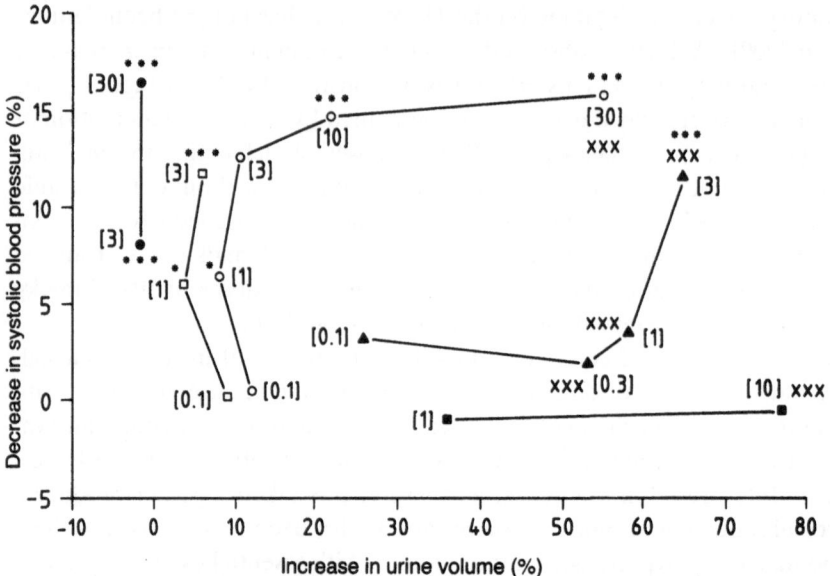

Fig. 48. Contrast of antihypertensive and diuretic effects of cicletanine (o) after 2 weeks' treatment of spontaneously hypertensive rats of the stroke-prone strain. The *curves* for captopril (□), hydrochlorothiazide (■), indapamide (▲) and prazosine (•) are given for comparison. The *figures in brackets* represent the dose (mg/kg). Significance: *, ˣ P < 0.05; **, ˣˣ P < 0.01; ***, ˣˣˣ P < 0.001; * fall in blood pressure; ˣ increase in urine volume [30]

50 mg/day develops slowly and only attains its maximum after some 3 months, the remaining constant for up to over 2 years (Fig. 49) [99].

This good long-term result is to be attributed, inter alia, to the excellent tolerance for cicletanine. Interruptions of treatment because of undesirable side effects or subjectively unpleasant sensations proved unnecessary in these studies [25]. Meanwhile the blood pressure-reducing effet of cicletanine was confirmed in the first placebo-controlled double-blind study [130]. Stimulation of the renin-angiotensin-aldosterone system was not usually established in the treated patients, so that a purely diuretic effect of cicletanine as the cause of the blood pressure reduction seems rather unlikely. Rather, the results of the short-term pharmacological experiments point to stimulation of prostacyclin synthesis as a central factor for the clinical effects of this substance. However, at the present time data on prostacyclin metabolism during long-term treatment with cicletanine are still completely lacking, so that supplementary clinical studies will be required in the future to reveal the entire action potential of cicletanine in the treatment of hypertension on a

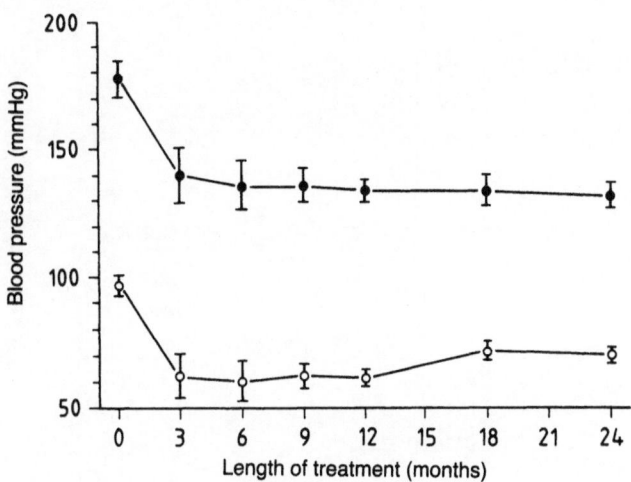

Fig. 49. Normalization of arterial blood pressure in 40 patients with mild primary hypertension during 2 years' treatment with 50 mg/day cicletanine. The values give the mean values ± standard deviation. The systolic blood pressure is represented by *closed symbols*, the diastolic pressure by *open symbols* [99]

firm basis. Certainly, the results of prospective studies over several years must be awaited to resolve the question whether it can ultimately exert an antiatherogenic, antithrombogenic and cardioprotective action by means of its prostacyclin-stimulating effect in a clinical setting.

To sum up, the stimulation of prostacyclin synthesis constitutes an attractive therapeutical principle in the management of hypertension aimed at compensating for a lack of endogenous prostacyclin in this condition. By virtue of the many-sided cellular actions of prostacyclin, this therapeutical principle may also possibly provide an opportunity for the simultaneous management of the complications of hypertension such as atherosclerosis with coronary heart disease, cerebral sclerosis and nephropathy. Hence, the stimulation of prostacyclin synthesis should be the object of further and more intensive research in the field of treatment of hypertension.

References

1. Abdel-Halim MS, Ekstedt J, Änggard E (1979) Determination of prostaglandin $F_{2\alpha}$, E_2, D_2 and 6-keto-$PGF_{1\alpha}$ in human cerebrospinal fluid, Prostaglandins 17: 405–409
2. Abdel-Halim MS, von Holst H, Meyerson B, Sachs C, Änggard E (1980) Prostaglandin profiles in tissue and blood vessels from human brain. J. Neurochem 34: 1331–1333
3. Abe K (1981) The kinins and prostaglandins in hypertension. Clin Endocrinol Metab 10: 577–605
4. Aiken JW, Gorman RR, Shebuski RJ (1979) Prevention of blockage of partially obstructed arteries with prostacyclin correlates with inhibition of platelet aggregation. Prostaglandins 17: 483–495
5. Araki H, Lefer AM (1980) Role of prostacyclin in the preservation of ischemic myocardial tissue in the perfused cat heart. Circ Res 47: 757–763
6. Armstrong JM, Lattimer N, Moncada S, Vane JR (1978) Comparison of the vasodepressor effects of prostacyclin and 6-oxo-prostaglandin $F_{1\alpha}$, with those of prostaglandin E_2 in rats and rabbits. Br J Pharmacol 62: 125–130
7. Axelrod L, Minnich AK, Ryan CA (1985) Stimulation of prostacyclin production in isolated rat adipocytes by angiotensin II, vasopressin, and bradykinin: Evidence for two separate mechanisms of prostaglandin synthesis. Endocrinology 116: 2548–2553
8. Baenziger NL, Becherer PR, Majerus PW (1979) Characterization of prostacyclin synthesis in cultures human arterial smooth muscle cells venous endothelial cells and skin fibroblasts. Cell 16: 967–974
9. Baenziger NL, Force LE, Becherer PR (1980) Histamine stimulates prostacyclin synthesis in cultured human umbilical vein endothelial cells. Biomed Biophys Res Commun 92: 1435–1440
10. Baenziger NL, Fogerty FJ, Mertz LF, Chernuta LF (1981) Regulation of histamine-mediated prostacyclin synthesis in cultured human vascular endothelial cells. Cell 24: 915–923
11. Barnett AH, Wakelin K, Leatherdale BA (1984) Specific thromboxane synthetase inhibition and albumin excretion rate in insulin-dependent diabetes. Lancet I: 1322–1325
12. Beckmann ML, Gerber JG, Byyny RL, LoVerde M, Nies AS (1988) Propranolol increases prostacyclin synthesis in patients with essential hypertension. Hypertension 12: 582–588
13. Beilin LJ, Bhattacharya J (1977) The effect of prostaglandin synthesis inhibitors on renal blood flow distribution in conscious rabbits. J Physiol 269: 395–405

14. Beitz J, Förster W (1980) Influence of human low density and high density lipoprotein cholesterol on the in vitro prostaglandin I_2 synthease activity. Biochim Biophys Acta 620: 352–355

15. Belch JJF, Cormie J, Newman P et al. (1983) Dazoxiben, a thromboxane synthetase inhibitor, in the treatment of Raynauds syndrome: a double-blind trial. Br J Clin Pharmacol 15 (Suppl 1): 113s–116s

16. Belch JJF, Saniabadi A, Dickson R, Sturrock RD, Forbes CD (1987) Effect of iloprost (ZK 36374) on white cell behavior. In: Gryglewski RJ, Stock G (eds) Prostacyclin and its stable analogue iloprost. Springer, Berlin Heidelberg New York Tokyo, pp 97–102

17. Bergman G, Atkinson L, Richardson PJ, Daly K, Rothman M, Jackson G, Jewitt DE (1981) Prostacyclin: Haemodynamic and metabolic effects in patients with coronary artery disease. Lancet I: 569–572

18. Bergström S, Ryhage R, Samuelsson B, Sjövall J (1962) The structure of prostaglandin E, F_1, and F_2. Acta Chem Scand 16: 501–502

19. Bönner G, Beck D, Deeg M, Marin-Grez M, Gross F (1982) Effects of frusemide on the renal kallikrein-kinin system of the rat. Clin Sci 63: 447–453

20. Botha JH, Leary WP, Asmal AC (1980) Enhanced release of a "prostacyclinlike" substance from aortic strips of spontaneously hypertensive rats. Prostaglandins 19: 285–289

21. Bourgain RH, Deby C, Andries R, Garay R, Braquet P (1984) The effect of cicletanin, a diuretic, on the platelet vessel wall interaction; its involvement in the arachidonic acid cascade. Biochem Pharmacol 33: 3917–3918

22. Bourgain RH, Deby C (1988) Enhancement of prostacyclin generation by cicletanine. Drugs Exptl Clin Res XIV: 135–139

23. Bourgain R (1989) Enhancement of prostacyclin/thromboxane A_2 ratio by cicletanine. Vortrag auf dem Kongreß über Prostacyclin-Synthese-Stimulation in der Hochdrucktherapie. Köln, 25. 2. 1989

24. Bouthier JA, Safar ME, Deschamps E, Tarrade T (1988) Hemodynamic effects of an antihypertensive duiretic substance on the forearm circulation of patients with essential hypertension. Drugs Exp Clin Res 14: 221–224

25. Bunting S, Gryglewski R, Moncada S, Vane JR (1976) Arterial walls generate from prostaglandin endoperoxides a substance (prostaglandin X) which relaxes strips of mesenteric and coeliac arteries and inhibits platelet aggregation. Prostaglandins 12: 897–913

26. Bursch W, Schulte-Hermann R (1987) Cytoprotective effect of iloprost against liver cell death induced by carbon tetrachloride (CCe4) or bromobenzene. In: Gryglewski RJ, Stock G (eds) Prostacyclin and its stable analogue iloprost. Springer, Berlin Heidelberg New York Tokyo, pp 257–268

27. Bush A, Busst C, Knight WB, Shineborune EA (1987) Modification of pulmonary hypertension secondary to congential heart disease by prostacyclin therapy. Am Rev Respir Dis 136: 767–769

28. Cahn J, Borzeix MG (1987) Iloprost in experimental cerebral ischemia. In: Gryglewski RJ, Stock G (eds) Prostacyclin and its stable analogue iloprost. Springer, Berlin Heidelberg New York Tokyo, pp 247–256

29. Campbell WB, Holland OB, Adams BV, Gomez-Sanchez CE (1982) Urinary excretion of prostaglandin E_2, prostaglandin $F_{2\alpha}$, and thromboxane B_2 in normotensive and hypertensive subjects on varying sodium intakes. Hypertension 4: 735–741

30. Chabrier PE, Guinot P, Tarrade T (1988) Cicletanine. Cardiovas Drug Rev 6: 166–179

31. Chang WC, Nakao J, Orimo H, Murota SI (1980) Stimulation of prostacyclin biosynthetic activity by estradiol in rat aortic smooth muscle cells in culture. Biochim Biophys Acta 619: 107–118

32. Chelly JE, Fabiani JN, Tricot AM, Abry B, Carpentier A (1987) Vasodilator properties of prostacyclin after coronary artery bypass surgery. J Cardiovasc Pharmacol 9: 142–147

33. Christ-Hazelhof E, Nugteren DH (1981) Prostacyclin is not a circulating hormone. Prostaglandins 22: 739–746

34. Chrysant SG, Townsend SM, Morgan PR (1978) The effects of salt and meclofenamate administration on the hypertension of spontaneously hypertensive rats. Clin Exp Hypertens 1: 381–391

35. Cinotti GA, Pierucci A, Ciabattoni G, Pugliese F, Simonetti BM, Patrono C (1982) Effects of prostacyclin infusion in man. In: Matero F, Biglieri EG, Edwards CRW (eds) Serono Symposium No. 50, "Endocrinology of hypertension". Academic Press, London New York, pp 333–336

36. Clair RWST (1976) Metbolism of the arterial wall and atherosclerosis. Atheroscler Rev 1: 61–117

37. Clostre F, Etienne A (1988) General pharmacology of cicletanine. Drugs Exptl Clin Res XIV: 73–82

38. Coceani F, Olley PM, Lock JE (1980) Prostaglandins, ductus arteriosus, pulmonary circulation: Current concepts and clinical potential. Eur J Clin Pharmacol 18: 75–81

39. Codde JP, Beilin LJ, Croft KD, Vandongen R (1987) Effects of altered prostanoid and lyso-PAF synthesis by marine oil diets on blood pressure of salt loaded spontaneously hypertensive rats. In: Bönner G, Carretero OA, Küppers H, McGiff JC (eds) Vasodepressor hormones in hypertension: Prostaglandins and kallikrein-kinins. Birkhäuser, Basel Boston, pp 101–110

40. Colina-Chourio JA, McGiff JC, Miller MP, Nasjletti A (1976) Possible influence of intrarenal generation of kinins on prostaglandin release from the rabbit perfused kidney. Br J Pharmacol 58: 165–172

41. Comberg HU, Heyden S, Hames CG, Vergroesen AJ, Fleischmann AI (1978) Hypotensive effect of dietary prostaglandin precursor in hypertensive man. Prostaglandins 15: 193–197

42. Corey EJ, Niwa H, Falck JR, Mioskowski C, Araiu Y, Marfat A (1980) Recent studies on the chemical synthesis of eicosanoids. Adv Prostagland Thrombox Leukotr Res 6: 19–23

43. Coughlin SR, Moskowitz MA, Zetter BR, Antoniades HN, Levine L (1980) Platelet-dependent stimulation of prostacyclin synthesis by platelet-derived growth factor. Nature 288: 600–602

44. Crutchley DJ, Ryan JW, Ryan US, Fisher GH (1983) Bradykinin-induced release of prostacyclin and thromboxanes from bovine pulmonary artery endothelial cells. Studies with lower homologs and calcium antagonists. Biochim Biophys Acta 751: 99–107

45. Darius H, Hossmann V, Schrör K (1986) Antiplatelet effects of intravenous iloprost in patients with peripheral arterial obliterative disease. A placebo-controlled dose-response study. Klin Wochenschr 64: 545–551

46. Data JL, Gerber JG, Crump WJ, Frölich JC, Hollifield JW, Nies A (1978) The prostaglandin system: A role in baroreceptor control of renin release. Circ Res 42: 454–458

47. Dembinska-Kiéc A, Rücker W, Schönhöfer PS (1979) Atherosclerosis decreased prostacyclin formation in rabbit lungs and kidneys. Prostaglandins 17: 831–839

48. DeWitt DL, Smith WL (1983) Purification of prostacyclin synthetase from bovine aorta by immunoaffinity chromatography. J Biol Chem 258: 3285–3293

49. Dietlein M, Lauster F, Scherer B (1988) Glomeruläre Filtrationsrate und renale Prostaglandine nach Eiweißzufuhr bei chronischer Niereninsuffizienz. Klin Wochenschr 66 (Suppl XIII): 194

50. Dorian B, Larrue J, Defeudis FV, Salari H, Borgeat P, Braquet P (1984) Activation of prostacyclin synthesis in cultured smooth muscle cells by diuretic antihypertensive drugs. Biochem Pharmacol 33: 2265–2269

51. Dorian B, Daret D, Braquet P, Larrue J (1988) Cicletanine and eicosanoids in cultered vascular smooth muscle cells. Drugs Exptl Clin Res XIV: 117–122

52. Düsing R, Scherhag R, Glänzer K, Budde U, Kramer HJ (1983) Dietary linoleic acid deprivation: Effects on blood pressure and PGI_2 synthesis. Am J Physiol 244: H228–H233

53. Düsing R, Pietsch R, Landsberg G, Scherf H, Glänzer K, Mutscher E, Kramer HJ (1986) Untersuchungen zur extrarenalen Wirkung von Diuretika. In: Krück F, Schrey A (Hrsg) Diuretika III. Springer, Berlin Heidelberg New York Tokyo, pp 38–45

54. Dunn MJ, Hood VL (1977) Prostaglandins and the kidney. Am J Physiol 233: F-169–F-184

55. Durao V, Prata MM, Goncalvez LMP (1977) Modification of antihypertensive effect of β-adrenoceptor blocking agents by inhibition of endogenous prostaglandin synthesis. Lancet II: 1005–1007

56. Dusting GJ, Moncada S, Vane JR (1978) Disappearance of prostacyclin (PGI_2) in the circulation of the dog. Brit J Pharmacol 62: 414P–415P

57. Ehnholm C, Huttunen J, Pietinen P, Leino U, Mutanen M, Kostianinen E, Pikkarainen J, Dougherty R, Iacono J, Puska P (1982) Effect of diet on serum lipoproteins in a population with a high risk of coronary heart disease. N Engl J Med 307: 850–855

58. Eldor A, Falcone DJ, Hajjar DP, Minick CR, Weksler BB (1981) Recovery of prostacyclin production by de-endothelialized rabbit aorta. J Clin Invest 67: 735–741

59. Eldor A, Falcone DJ, Hajjar DP, Minick CR, Weksler BB (1982) Diet-induced hypercholesterolemia inhibits the recovery of prostacyclin production by injured rabbit aorta. Am J Pathol 107: 186–190

60. Epstein M, Lifschitz M, Rappaport K (1982) Augmentation of prostaglandin production by linoleic acid in man. Clin Sci 63: 565–571

61. Euler US von (1934) Zur Kenntnis der pharmakologischen Wirkungen von Nativsekreten und Extrakten männlicher accessorischer Geschlechtsdrüsen. Naunyn-Schmiedebergs Arch Pharmacol 175: 78–84

62. Euler US von (1935) Über die spezifische blutdrucksenkende Substanz des menschlichen Prostata- und Samenblasensekretes. Klin Wochenschr 14: 1182–1183

63. Evensen SA (1979) Injury to cultured endothelial cells. The role of lipoproteins and thrombo-active agents. Haemostasis 8: 203–210

64. Falardeau P, Martineau A (1983) In vivo production of prostaglandin I_2 in Dahl salt-sensitive and salt-resistant rats. Hypertension 5: 701–705

65. Favre L, Glasson PH, Riondel A, Vallotton MB (1983) Interaction of diuretics and nonsteroidal anti-inflammatory drugs in man. Clin Sci 64: 407–412

66. Favre L, Vallotton MB (1984) Relationship of renal prostaglandins to three diuretics. Prostagland Leukotr Med. 14; 313–319

67. Fitzgerald DJ, Entman SS, Mulloy K, FitzGerald GA (1987) Decreased prostacyclin biosynthesis preceding the clinical manifestation of pregnancy-induced hypertension. Circulation 75: 856–963

68. FitzGerald GA, Hossmann V, Hummerich W, Konrads A (1980) The renin-kallikrein-prostaglandin system: Plasma active and inactive renin and urinary kallikrein during prostacyclin infusion in man. Prostagland Med 5: 445–456

69. FitzGerald GA, Brash AR, Falardeau P, Oates JA (1981) Estimated rate of prostacyclin secretion into the circulation of normal man. J Clin Invest 68: 1272–1276

70. Fleisher LN, Tall AR, Witte LD, Miller RW, Cannon PJ (1981) Stimulation of arterial endothelial cell prostacyclin synthesis by high density lipoproteins. Circulation 64: IV–216

71. Flower RJ, Cardinal DC (1979) Use of a novel platelet aggregometer to study the generation by, and actions of prostacyclin in whole blood. In: Vane JR, Bergström S (eds) Prostacyclin. Raven Press, New York, pp 211–220

72. Fodor GP, Guinot P (1988) Review of three studies to determine the efficacy and tolerance of cicletanine in the short- and long-term treatment of essential hypertension. Drug Exp Clin Res 14: 195–204

73. Förster W (1980) Effect of various agents on prostaglandin biosynthesis and the antiaggregatory effect. Acta Med Scand Suppl 642: 35–46

74. Frey EK, Kraut H (1926) Über einen von der Niere ausgeschiedenen, die Herztätigkeit anregenden Stoff. Hoppe-Seylers Z Physiol Chem 157: 32–61

75. Friedman LA, Webster J, Hensby CN, Lewsi PJ (1981) Prostacyclin production in arterial hypertension. In: Lewis PJ, O'Grady J (eds) Clinical pharmacology of prostacyclin. Raven Press, New York, pp 97–102

76. Frölich JC, Hollifield JW, Dormois JC (1976) Suppression of plasma renin activity by indomethacin in man. Circ Res 39: 447–452

77. Frölich JC, Hollifield JW, Vesper BS, Shand DG, Wilson JP, Seyberth HJ, Frölich WH, Oates JA (1979) Reduction of plasma renin activity by inhibition

of the fatty acid cyclooxygenase: Independence of sodium retention. Circ Res 44: 781–787

78. Frölich JC, Robertson D, Kitajima W, Rosenkranz B, Reimann I (1981) Prostaglandins in human hypertension: Relationship to renin, sodium, and antihypertensive drug action. In: Laragh JH, Bühler F, Seldin DW (eds) Frontiers in hypertension research. Springer, New York, pp 114–118

79. Frölich JC, Rosenkranz B (1982) Role of prostaglandins in the regulation of blood pressure. In: Hermann AG, Vanhoute PM, Denolin H, Goossens A (eds) Cardiovascular pharmacology of the prostaglandins. Raven Press, New York, pp 259–265

80. Galler M, Folkert VW, Schlondorff D (1981) Effect of converting enzyme inhibitor on prostaglandin synthesis by isolated rat glomeruli. Clin Res 29: 271A

81. Gant NF, Daley GL, Chand S, Whorley RJ, MacDonald PC (1973) A study of angiotensin II pressor response throughout primigravid pregnancy. J Clin Invest 52: 2682–2689

82. Garay R, Hornych A, Juin G, Nazaret C, Hannaert P, Deschamps de Paillette E, Braquet P (183) K^+-transport, membrane potential and the AA cascade in the vasodilator antihypertensive effects of cicletanide. II. Clinical aspect. Naunyn Schmiedebergs Arch Pharmacol 324 (Suppl): 240

83. Gbeassor FM, Grose JM, Lebel M (1982) Effects of indapamide on prostaglandins synthesis. Clin Invest Med 5: 26B

84. Gerber JC, Payne NA, Murphy RC, Nies AS (1981) Prostacyclin produced by the pregnant uterus in the dog may act as a circulating vasodepressor substance. J Clin Invest 67: 632–636

85. Glänzer K, Prüßing B, Düsing R, Kramer HJ (1982) Hemodynamic and hormonal responses to 8-arginine-vasopressin in healthy man: Effects of indomethacin. Klin Wochenschr 60: 1234–1239

86. Goehlert UG, Ng Ying Kin NMK, Wolfe LS (1981) Biosynthesis of prostacyclin in rat cerebral microvessels and the choroid plexus. J Neurochem 36: 1192–1201

87. Goldblatt MW (1935) Properties of human seminal plasma. J Physiol 84: 208–218

88. Goldstone R, Martin K, Zipser R, Horton R (1981) Evidence for a dual action converting enzyme inhibitor on blood pressure in normal man. Prostaglandins 2: 587–598

89. Gorman RR, Bunting S, Miller OV (1977) Modulation of human platelet adenylate cyclase by prostacyclin (PGX). Prostaglandins 13: 377–388

90. Gothberg G, Lundin S, Folkow B (1982) Acute vasodepressor effect in normotensive rats following extracorporal perfusion of the declipped kidney of two-kidney/one-clip hypertensive rats. Hypertension 4, Suppl II: 101–105

91. Grodzinska L, Basista M, Basista E, Slawinski M, Swies J, Stachura J, Ohlrogge R (1987) Nitrendipine-stimulated release of prostacyclin-like substance in normal and atherosclerotic animals. Arzneimittelforsch 37: 412–415

92. Grose JH, Lebel M, Gbeassor FM (1980) Diminished urinary prostacyclin metabolite in essential hypertension Clin Sci 59: 121s–123s

93. Grose JH, Lebel M, Gbeassor FM (1982) Abnormal urinary 6-keto-prostaglandin $F_{1\alpha}$ and thromboxane B_2 in essential hypertension. Clin Invest Med 5: 2–3

94. Gryglewski RJ, Bunting S, Moncada S, Flower RJ, Vane JR (1976) Arterial walls are protected against deposition of platelet thrombi by a substance (pro-staglandin X) which they make from prostaglandin endoperoxides. Prostaglan-dins 12: 685–713

95. Gryglewski RJ, Dembinska-Kiéc A, Zmuda A, Gryglewska T (1978) Prostacy-clin and thromboxane A_2 biosynthesis capacities of heart, arteries and platelets at various stages of experimental atherosclerosis in rabbits. Atherosclerosis 31: 385–394

96. Gryglewski RJ, Korbut R, Ocetkiewicz A (1978) De-aggregatory action of pro-stacyclin in vivo and its enhancement by theophylline. Prostaglandins 15: 637–644

97. Gryglewski RJ, Korbut R, Ocetkiewicz A (1978) Generation of prostacyclin by lungs in vivo and its release into the arterial circulation. Nature 273: 765–767

98. Guinot P, Frölich JC (1985) Study of the effects of cicletanine on prostanoids. Arzneimittelforschung 35: 1714–1716

99. Guinot P, Jewitt-Harris J, Tarrade T (1989) Determination of the optimal dose of the antihypertensive drug cicletanine hydrochloride in man. Drug Res 39: 86–89

100. Gullner HG, Cerletti C,Bartter FC, Smith JB, Gill JR (1979) Prostacyclin over-production in Bartter's syndrome. Lancet II: 767–769

101. Gullner HG, Nicolaou KC, Bartter FC (1980) Prostacyclin has effects on prox-imal and distal tubular function in the dog. Prostagland Med 6: 141–146

102. Haberey M, Loge O, Maaß B, Ohme G (1987) Hemodynamic profile of iloprost in rats, rabbits and cats. In: Gryglewski RJ, Stock G (eds) Prostacyclin and its stable analogue iloprost. Springer, Berlin Heidelberg New York Tokyo, pp 151–158

103. Hajjar DP, Weksler BB, Falcone DJ, Hefton JM, Tackgoldman K, Minick CR (1982) Prostacyclin modulates cholesteryl ester hydrolytic activity by its effect on cyclic adenosine monophosphate in rabbit aortic smooth muscle cells. J Clin Invest 70: 479–488

104. Hajjar DP (1984) Prostacyclin and cyclic nucleotides interact to modulate arterial cholesteryl ester metabolism. In: Greengard P et al. (eds) Advances in cyclic nucleotide and protein phosphorylation research, Vol 17. Raven Press, New York, pp 605–614

105. Hajjar DP (1985) Prostaglandins and cyclic nucleotides. Modulators of arterial cholesterol metabolism. Biomed Pharmacol 34: 295–300

106. Ham EA, Egan RW, Sodermann DD, Gale PH, Kuehl Jr FA (1979) Peroxidase-dependent deactivation of prostacyclin synthetase. J Biol Chem 254: 2191–2194

107. Hanley SP, Cockbill SR, Bevan J, Hepinstall S (1981) Differential inhibition by low dose aspirin of human venous prostacyclin synthesis and platelet thrombo-xane synthesis. Lancet II: 969–971

108. Harold JG, Siegel RJ, FitzGerald GA, Satoh P, Fishbein MC (1988) Differential prostacyclin production by human umbilical vasculature. Arch Pathol Lab Med 112: 43–46

109. Hassid A, Williams C (1983) Vasoconstrictor-evoked prostaglandin synthesis in cultured vascular smooth muscle. Am J Physiol 245: C278–C282

110. Haslam RJ, Davidson MML, Fox JEB, Lynham JA (1978) Cyclic nucleotides in platelet function. Thromb Haemost 40: 232–240

111. Haslam RJ, McClemaghan MD (1981) Measurement of circulating prostacyclin. Nature 292: 364–366

112. Hawiger J, Parkinson S, Timmons S (1980) Prostacyclin inhibits mobilization of fibrinogen binding sites on human ADP and thrombin treated platelets. Nature 283: 195–197

113. Henriksson P, Edhag O, Wennmalm A (1985) Prostacyclin infusion in patients with acute myocardial infarction. Br Heart J 53: 173–179

114. Hensby CN (1981) Plasma 6-Oxo-PGF$_{1\alpha}$ in man. In: Lewis PJ, O'Grady J (eds) Clinical pharmacology of prostacyclin. Raven Press, New York, pp 37–44

115. Hermiller JB, Bambach D, Thompson MJ, Huss P, Fontana ME, Magorien RD, Unverferth DV, Leier CV (1982) Vasodilators and prostaglandin inhibitors in primary pulmonary hypertension. Ann Intern Med 97: 480–489

116. Higenbottam T (1987) The place of prostacyclin in the clinical management of primary pulmonary hypertension. Am Rev Respir Dis 136: 785–788

117. Hojvat SA, Musch MW, Miller RJ (1983) Stimulation of prostaglandin production in rabbit ileal mucosa by bradykinin. J Pharmacol Exp Ther 226: 749–755

118. Honda M, Manabe R, Minato M, Watanabe M, Fukuda N, Izumi Y, Hatano M (1986) Effects of intravenous administration of a calcium antagonist on prostaglandins and thromboxane in plasma and urine in humans. Prostagland Leuk Med 23: 289–302

119. Hong SL, Levine L (1976) Stimulation of prostaglandin synthesis by bradykinin and thrombin and their mechanisms of action on MC 5–5 fibroblasts. J Biol Chem 251: 5814–5816

120. Hong SL (1980) Effect of bradykinin and thrombin on prostacyclin synthesis in endothelial cells from calf and pig aorta and human umbilical cord vein. Thromb Res 18: 787–795

121. Hope W, Martin TJ, Chesterman CN, Morgan FJ (1979) Human β-thromboglobulin inhibits PGI$_2$ production and binds to a specific site in bovine aortic endothelial cells. Nature 282: 210–212

122. Hornych A, Safar M, Bariety J, Simon A, London G, Levenson J (1983) Thromboxane B$_2$ in borderline and essential hypertensive patients. Prostagland Leukotr Med 10: 145–155

123. Ipsen (1987) Tenstaten (Ciclétanine). Dossier scientifique á l'usage de MM. les experts.

124. Jeremy JY, Barradas MA, Mikhailidis DP, Dandona P (1985) An investigation into the effects of nifedipine and nimodipine on platelet function and vascular prostacyclin synthesis. Drug Exp Clin Res 11: 645–651

125. Johnson M, Harrison HE, Raftery AT, Elder JB (1981) Prostacyclin and diabetes. In: Lewis PJ, O'Grady J (eds) Clinical pharmacology of prostacyclin. Raven Press, New York, pp 105–112

126. Johnson RA, Morton DR, Kinner JH, Gorman RR, McGuire JC, Sun FF (1976) The chemical structure of prostaglandin X (prostacyclin). Prostaglandins 12: 915–928

127. Jones DK, Higenbottam TW, Wallwork J (1987) Treatment of primary pulmonary hypertension with intravenous epoprostenol (prostacyclin). Br Heart J 57: 270–278

128. Jouve R, Langlet F, Puddu PE, Rolland PH, Guillen JC, Cano JP, Serradimigni A (1986) Cicletanide improves outcome after left circumflex coronary artery occlusion-reperfusion in the dog. J Cardiovase Pharmacol 8: 208–215

129. Jouve R, Puddu PE, Langlet F, Lanti M, Guillen JC, Rolland PH, Serradi-Migni A (1988) Effects of cicletanine in the left circumflex coronary artery occlusion-reperfusion canine model of sudden death: Analysis of 107 experiments using Cox's proportional hazards model. Drug Exp Clin Res 14: 167–180

130. Jungers P (1989) Cicletanin in the elderly hyperntensive patients. Vortrag auf dem Kongreß über Prostacyclin-Synthese-Stimulation in der Hochdrucktherapie. Köln, 25. 2. 1989. In: Tarrade T, Forette F, Jungers P, Mettelus I (1989) Efficacite et tolerance du cicletanine chez le sujet age. Hypertendu, Therapie 44 (im Druck)

131. Kahlen I, Schrör K (1982) Mepindolol protection of prostacyclin formation. Subsequent increase in arachidonic acid-induced prostacyclin release in isolated guinea pig heart. Eur J Pharmacol 82: 81–84

132. Kelton J, Carter C, Buchanan MR, Hirsh J (1978) Thrombogenic effect of high dose aspirin in injury-induced experimental venous thrombosis (abstr). Clin Res 26: 350A

133. Kelton JG, Blajchman MA (1980) Prostaglandin I$_2$ (prostacyclin). Can Med Assoc J 122: 175–179

134. Kulkarni PS, Roberts R, Needleman P (1976) Paradoxical endogenous synthesis of a coronary dilating substance from arachidonate. Prostaglandins 12: 337–353

135. Kurzrock R, Lieb CC (1930) Biochemical studies of human semen. II. The action of semen on the human uterus. Proc Soc Exp Biol Med 28: 268–272

136. Lamas CJ, Lamas C (1977) Prostaglandin metabolism in the kidneys of spontaneously hypertensive rats. Am J Physiol 233: H87–H92

137. Larrson C, Weber P, Änggard E (1974) Arachidonic acid increases and indomethacin decreases plasma renin activity in the rabbit. Europ J Pharmacol 28: 391–394

138. Larrue J, Rigaud M, Daret D, Demond J, Durrand J, Bricaud H (1980) Prostacyclin production by cultured smooth muscle cells from atherosclerotic rabbit aorta. Nature 285: 480–483

139. Larrue J, Leroux C, Daret D, Bricaud H (1982) Decreased prostaglandin production in cultured smooth muscle cells from atherosclerotic rabbit aorta. Biochim Biophys Acta 710: 257–263

140. Latta G, Schrör K (1988) Kalziumantagonisten und Thrombozytenfunktion. Hämostaseologie 8: 80–89

141. Lebel M, Grose JH (1982) Renal prostaglandins in borderline and sustained essential hypertension. Prostagland Leukotr Med 8: 409–418

142. Lebel M, Grose JH, Belleau LJ, Langlois S (1983) Effects of indapamide on renal prostaglandin production in hypertensive patients. Curr Med Res Opin 2: 81–86

143. Lefer AM, Ogletree ML, Smith JB, Silver MJ, Nicolaou KC, Barnette WE, Gasic GP (1978) Prostacyclin: A potentially valuable agent for preserving myocardial tissue in acute myocardial ischemia. Science 200: 52–56

144. Levin RI, Jaffe EA, Weksler BB, Tackgoldman K (1981) Nitroglycerin stimulates synthesis of prostacyclin by cultured human endothelial cells. J Clin Invest 67: 762–769

145. Levine L, Moskowitz MA (1979) α- and β-adrenergic stimulation of arachidonic acid metabolism in cells in culture. Proc Natl Acad Sci 76: 6632–6636

146. Levy J (1977) Changes in systolic arterial blood pressure in normal and spontaneously hypertensive rats produced by acute administration of inhibitors of prostaglandin biosynthesis. Prostaglandins 13: 153–160

147. Locher RA, Block LH, Tenschert W, Vetter W (1982) Interaction of vasopressin and prostaglandin in human monocytes. In: Matero F, Biglieri EG, Edwards CRW (eds) Serono Symposium No. 50, "Endocrinology of hypertension". Academic Press, London New York, pp 325–332

148. Lock JF, Olley PM, Coceam F, Swyer PR, Row RD (1979) Use of prostacyclin persistent fetal circulation. Lancet I: 1343

149. Lonchampt MO, Marche P, Demerle C (1988) Histamin H_1-receptors mediate phophoinositide and calcium response in cultured smooth muscle cells. Interactions with cicletanine. Agents Actions 24: 255–260

150. Long WA, Rubin LJ (1987) Prostacyclin and PGE treatment of pulmonary hypertension. Am Rev Respir Dis 136: 773–776

151. Lopez-Ovejero JA, Weber MA, Drayer JIM, Sealy JE, Laragh JH (1978) Effects of indomethacin alone and during diuretic or β-adrenoreceptor-blockade therapy on blood pressure and the renin system in essential hypertension. Clin Sci Mol Med 55: 203s–205s

152. Lorenz R, Spengler U, Fischer S, Duhm J, Weber P (1983) Platelet function, thromboxane formation and blood pressure control during supplementation of the western diet with cod liver oil. Circulation 67: 504–511

153. Lukaesko P, Messina EJ, Kaley G (1980) Reduced hypotensive action of arachidonic acid in the spontaneously hypertensive rat. Hypertension 2: 657–663

154. MacIntyre DE, Pearson JD, Gordon JL (1978) Localisation and stimulation of prostacyclin production in vascular cells. Nature 271: 549–551

155. MacNab MW, Foltz EL, Graves BS, Rinehart RK, Tripp SL, Feliciano NR, Sen S (1984) The effects of a new thromboxane synthetase inhibitor, CGS-13080, in man. J Clin Pharmacol 24: 76–83

156. Malherbe ES, Le Hegarat M, Baranes J, Clostre F, Braquet P (1988) Comparison of cicletanine with other antihypertensive drugs in SHR-SP models. Drug Exp Clin Res 14: 83–88

157. Marche P, Girard A (1988) Phosphoinositides and cicletanine. Drugs Exptl Clin Res XIV: 103–108

158. Martineau A, Robillard M, Falardeau P (1983) Defective synthesis of vasodilator prostaglandins in the spontaneously hypertensive rat. Hypertension 6: I-161–I-165

159. Masotti G, Pogessi L, Galanti G, Trotta F, Neri Serneri GG (1981) Prostacyclin production in man. In: Lewis PJ, O'Grady J (eds) Clinical pharmacology of prostacyclin. Raven Press, New York, pp 9–20

160. Matzky R, Darius H, Schrör K (1982) The release of prostacyclin (PGI_2) by pentoxifylline from human vascular tissue. Arzneimittelforschung 32: 1315–1318
161. McGiff JC, Crowshaw K, Itskovitz HD (1974) Prostaglandins and renal function. Fed Proc 33: 39–47
162. McGiff JC, Nasjletti A (1976) Kinins, renal function and blood pressure regulation. Fred Proc 35: 172–174
163. McGiff JC, Wong PY-K (1979) Compartimentalization of prostaglandin and prostacyclin within the kidney: Implications for renal function. Fed Proc 38: 89–93
164. McGiff JC (1980) Interactions of prostaglandins with the kallikrein-kinin and renin-angiotensin systems. Clin Sci 59: 105s–116s
165. McGowan HM, Vandongen R, Codde JP, Croft KD (1986) Increased aortic PGI_2 and plasma lyso-PAF in the unclipped one-kidney hypertensive rat. Am J Physiol 251: H1361–H1364
166. Mehta J, Metha P, Ostrowski N (1986) Calcium blocker diltiazem inhibits platelet activation and stimulates vascular prostacyclin synthesis. Am J Med Sci 291: 20–24
167. Miller OV, Gorman RR (1979) Evidence of distinct prostaglandin I_2 and D_2 receptors in human platelets. J Pharmacol Exp Ther 210: 134–140
168. Mills DCB, Smith JB (1971) The influence on platelet aggregation of drugs that affect the accumulation of adenosine 3', 5'cyclic monophosphate in platelets. Biochem J 121: 185–196
169. Moncada S, Gryglewski RJ, Bunting S, Vane JR (1976) A lipid peroxide inhibits the enzyme in blood vessel microsomes that generates from prostaglandin endoperoxides the substance (prostaglandin X) which prevents platelet aggregation. Prostaglandins 12: 715–733
170. Moncada S, Herman AG, Vane H (1977) Differential formation of prostacyclin (PGX or PGI_2) by layers of the arterial wall. An explanation for the antithrombotic properties of vascular endothelium. Thromb Res 11: 323–344
171. Moncada S, Higgs EGA, Vane JR (1977) Human arterial and venous tissues generate prostacyclin (prostaglandin X), a potent inhibitor of platelet aggregation. Lancet I: 18–21
172. Moncada S, Vane JR (1977) The discovery of prostacyclin – a fresh insight into arachidonic acid metabolism. In: Kharasch N, Fried J (eds) Biochemical aspects of prostaglandins and thromboxanes. Academic Press, New York, pp 155–177
173. Moncada S, Korbut R, Bunting S, Vane JR (1978) Prostacyclin is a circulating hormone. Nature 273: 767–777
174. Moncada S, Vane JR (1979) Arachidonic acid metabolites and the interactions between platelets and blood-vessel walls. E Engl J Med 300: 1142–1147
175. Moncada S (1982) Biological importance of prostacyclin. Br J Pharmacol 76: 3–31
176. Moncada S, Higgs EA (1986) Arachidonate metabolism in blood cells and the vessel wall. Clin Haematol 15: 273–292
177. Moore TJ, Crantz FR, Hollenberg NK, Koletsky RJ, Leboff MS, Swartz SL, Levine L, Podolsky S, Dluhy RG, Williams GH (1981) Contribution of prosta-

glandins to the antihypertensive action of captopril in essential hypertension. Hypertension 3: 168–173

178. Morera S, Santoro FM, Rosón MI, de la Riva IJ (1983) Prostacyclin (PGI$_2$) synthesis in the vascular wall of rats with bilateral renal artery stenosis. Hypertension 5: V-38–V-42

179. Mortensen JZ, Schmidt EB, Nielsen AH, Dyerberg J (1983) The effect of N-6 and N-3 polyunsaturated fatty acids on hemostasis, blood lipids and blood pressure. Thromb Haemost 50: 543–546

180. Müller B, Maaß B, Stürzebecher C-S, Witt W (1987) The effect of iloprost and infarct size after coronary artery ligation. In: Gryglewski RJ, Stock G (eds) Prostacyclin and its stable analogue iloprost. Springer, Berlin Heidelberg New York Tokyo, pp 195–204

181. Mullane KM, Moncada S (1980) Prostacyclin release and the modulation of some vasoactive hormones. Prostaglandins 20: 25–49

182. Nadler J, Zipser RD, Coleman R, Horton R (1983) Stimulation of renal prostaglandins by pressor hormones in man: Comparison of prostaglandin E$_2$ and Prostacyclin (6-keto-prostaglandin F$_{1\alpha}$). JCE & M 56: 1260–1265

183. Nadler JL, Frederich OL, Hsueh W, Horton R (1986) Evidence of prostacyclin deficiency in the syndrome of hyporeninemic hypoaldosteronism. New Engl J Med 314: 1015–1020

184. Nadler JL, McKay M, Campese V, Vrabanac J, Horton R (1986) Evidence that prostacyclin modulates the vascular actions of calcium in man. J Clin Invest 77: 1278–1284

185. Nakagawa M, Kitani T, Kawamura T, Maeda Y, Osamura K, Rin K, Ijichi H (1981) Prostacyclin generation of vessel wall during the development of hypertension and the effect of antihypertensive agents. VIII. International Congress of Pharmacology, Tokyo, July 19–24. Book of abstracts, p 846

186. Nakagawa M, Takamatsu H, Toyoda T, Sawada S, Tsuji H, Ijichi H (1987) Effect of inhibition of Na$^+$-K$^+$-ATPase on the prostacyclin generation of cultured human vascular endothelial cells. Life Sci 40: 351–357

187. Nakao J, Chang WC, Murato SI, Orimo H (1981) Testosterone inhibits prostacyclin production by rat aortic smooth muscle cells in culture. Atherosclerosis 39: 203–209

188. Needleman P, Wyche A, Raz A (1979) Platelet and blood vessel arachidonate metabolism and interactions. J Clin Invest 63: 345–349

189. Negus P, Tannen RL, Dunn J (1976) Indomethacin potentiates the vasoconstrictor actions of angiotensin II in normal man. Prostaglandins 12: 175–180

190. Norris PG, Jones CJH, Weston MY (1986) Effect of dietary supplementation with fish oil on systolic blood pressure in mild hypertension. Br Med J 293: 104–105

191. Nowak J, Wennalm A (1978) Influence of indomethacin and of prostaglandin E$_1$ on total and regional blood flow in man. Acta Physiol Scand 102: 484–491

192. Ogihara T, Maruyama A, Hata T, Mikami H, Nakamaru M, Naka T, Ohde H, Kumahara Y (1981) Hormonal responses to long-term converting enzyme inhibition in hypertensive patients. Clin Pharmacol Ther 30: 328–325

193. O'Grady J, Bunting S, Flower R, Warrington S, Moti MJ, Fowle ASE, Higgs EA, Moncada S (1980) Effects of intravenous infusion of prostacyclin (PGI$_2$) in man. Prostaglandins 19: 319–333

194. Ohde H, Ogihara T, Nakamaru M, Higaki J, Gotoh S, Masuo K, Ohtsuka A, Sacki S, Kumahara Y (1982) Effect of prostacyclin infusion on active and inactive renin release in the isolated perfused kidney. Life Sci 31: 3031–3035

195. Ohno T, Yajima T, Urano T, Nakamura K (1984) Interaction of prostaglandin E$_2$ and bradykinin in the induction of afferent splanchnic nerve discharges in cats. Jap J Pharmacol 34: 191–202

196. Okahara T, Imanishi M, Abe Y, Yamamoto K (1983) Renal prostaglandins (PGs) and thromboxanes (TXs) release induced by bradykinin. Adv Exp Med Biol 156A: 515–518

197. Okuma M, Yamori Y, Ohta K, Uchino H (1979) Production of prostacyclinlike substance in stroke-prone and stroke-resistant spontaneously hypertensive rats. Prostaglandins 17: 1–7

198. Oparil S, Horton R, Wilkins LH, Irvin J, Hammett DK (1987) Antihypertensive effect of enalapril in essential hypertension: Role of prostacyclin. Am J Med Sci 294: 395–402

199. Orekhov AN, Tertov VV, Smirnov VN (1983) Prostacyclin analogues as antiatherosclerotic drugs. Lancet II: 521

200. Overlack A, Stumpe KO, Kuehnert M, Kolloch R, Ressel C, Heck I, Krueck F (1981) Evidence for participation of kinins in the antihypertensive effect of converting enzyme inhibition. Klin Wochenschr 59: 69–74

201. Pace-Asciak CR (1976) Decreased renal prostaglandin catabolism precedes onset of hypertension in the developing spontaneously hypertensive rat. Nature 263: 510–512

202. Pace-Asciak CR, Rangaraj G (1978) Prostaglandin biosynthesis and catabolism in the lamb ductus arteriosus, aorta and pulmonary artery. Biochim Biophys Acta 529: 13–20

203. Pace-Asciak CR, Carrara MC, Nicolaou KC (1978) Prostaglandin I$_2$ has more potent hypotensive properties than prostaglandin E$_2$ in the normal and spontaneously hypertensive rat. Prostaglandins 15: 999–1003

204. Pace-Asciak CR, Carrara MC, Rangaraj G, Nicolaou KC (1978) Enhanced formation of PGI$_2$, a potent hypotensive substance, by aortic rings and homogenates of the spontaneously hypertensive rat. Prostaglandins 15: 1005–1013

205. Patah RV, Mookerjee BK, Bentzel CJ, Hysert PE, Babej M, Lee JB (1975) Antagonism of the effects of furosemide by indomethacin in normal and hypertensive man. Prostaglandins 10: 649–659

206. Patrono C, Pugliese F, Giabattoni G, Patrignani P, Maseri A, Chierchia S, Peskar BA, Cinotti GA, Simonetti BM, Pierucci A (1982) Evidence for a direct stimulatory effect of prostacyclin on renin release in man. J Clin Invest 69: 231–239

207. Pearson JD (1982) Plasma factors regulating prostaglandin biosynthesis and catabolism. In: Hermann AG, Van Houtte PM, Goosens A, Denolin H (eds) Prostaglandins and the cardiovascular system. Raven Press, New York, pp 24–33

208. Pierucci A, Simonetti M, Ciabattoni G, Taggi F, Morabito S, Vastano S, Pugliese F (1986) Effect of prostacyclin on renal kallikrein release in man. Eur J Clin Invest 16: 233–238

209. Piere R (1988) Dossier d'expertise pharmacologique d'A.M.M. Dossier no. 328747.9

210. Pifer DD, Cagen LM, Chesney CM (1981) Stability of prostaglandin I_2 in human blood. Prostaglandins 21: 165–175

211. Preston FF, Whipps S, Jackson GA, French AJ, Wyld PJ, Stoddard GJ (1981) Inhibition of prostacyclin and platelet thromboxane A_2 after low dose aspirin. N Engl J Med 402: 76–79

212. Puska P, Nissinen A, Vartiainen E, Dougherty R, Multanen M, Iacono JM, Leino U, Korhonen HJ, Pietinen P, Moisio S (1983) Controlled, randomised trial of the effect of dietary fat on blood pressure. Lancet I: 1–5

213. Puustinen T, Uotila P (1983) The effect of bradykinin, histamine, and leukotrienes B_4, C_4 and D_4 on the formation of 6-keto-prostaglandin $F_{1\alpha}$ and thromboxane B_2 in hamster lungs. Prostagland Leukotr Med 12: 443–448

214. Quirion R, Rioux F, Regoli D (1978) The effect of an acute or chronic treatment with indomethacin on the blood pressure of DOCA/salt and spontaneously hypertensive rats. Clin Exp Hypertens 1: 267–277

215. Rademaker M, Thomas RHM, Provost G, Beacham JA, Cooke ED, Kirby JD (1987) Prolonged increase in digital blood flow following iloprost infusion in patients with systemic sclerosis. Postgrad Med J 63: 617–620

216. Rao RH, Rao UB, Srikantia SG (1981) Effect of polyunsaturate-rich vegetable oils on blood pressure in essential hypertension. Clin Exp Hypertens 3: 27–38

217. Rapp NS, Zenser TV, Mattammal MB, Davis BB (1981) Inhibition of bradykinin stimulation of renal medullary prostaglandin E_2 synthesis by phosphodiesterase inhibitors. J Pharmacol Exp Ther 219: 442–446

218. Rich S, Hart K, Kieras K, Brundage BH (1987) Thromboxane synthetase inhibition in primary pulmonary hypertension. Chest 91: 356–360

219. Richelsen B (1987) Factors regulating the production of prostaglandin E_2 and prostacyclin (prostaglandin I_2) in rat and human adipocytes. Biochem J 247: 389–394

220. Ritter JM, Barrow SE, Blair IA, Dollery CT (1983) Release of prostacyclin in vivo and its role in man. Lancet I: 317–319

221. Ritter JM, Hamilton G, Barrow SE, Heavey DJ, Hickling NE, Taylor KM, Hobbs KEF, Dollery CT (1986) Prostacyclin in the circulation of patients with vascular disorders undergoing surgery. Clin Sci 71: 743–747

222. Rosenkranz B, Fischer C, Weimer KE, Frölich JC (1980) Metabolism of prostacyclin and 6-keto-prostaglandin $F_{1\alpha}$ in man. J Biol Chem 255: 10194–10198

223. Rubin LJ, Groves BM, Reeves JT, Frosolono M, Handel F, Cato AE (1982) Prostacyclin-induced acute pulmonary vasodilation in primary pulmonary hypertension. Circulation 66: 334–338

224. Säynävälammi P (1986) Effects of captopril on the urinary excretion of prostanoids and kallikrein in spontaneously hypertensive rats. Acta Pharmacol Toxicol 59: 285–290

225. Säynävälammi P, Arvola P, Kulsmanen K, Seppälä E, Nurmi AK, Manninen V, Vapaatalo H (1987) Effects of indomethacin on hormonal and blood pressure responses to captopril in spontaneously hypertensive rats. Pharmacol Toxicol 61: 195–198

226. Säynävälammi P, Poersti I, Poesti P, Nurmi AK, Seppaelae E, Manninen V, Vapaatalo H (1988) Effects of the converting enzyme inhibitor quinapril (CI-906) on blood pressure, renin-angiotensin system, and prostanoids in essential hypertension. J Cardiovasc Pharmacol 12: 88–93

227. Salvetti A, Pedrinelli R (1982) Pharmacological evaluation of prostaglandins and their interaction with renin secretion in human hypertension. In: Mantero F, Biglieri EG, Edwards CRW (eds) Serono Symposium No. 50 "Endocrinology of hypertension". Academic Press, London New York, pp 243–256

228. Sanchez-Ramos L, O'Sullivan MJ, Garrido-Calderon J (1987) Effect of lowdose aspirin on angiotensin II pressor response in human pregnancy. Am J Obstet Gynecol 87: 193–194

229. Scherer B, Weber PC (1979) Time-dependent changes in prostaglandin excretion in response to furosemide in man. Clin Sci 56: 77–81

230. Schoeffer P, Ghysel-Burton R, Cabanie M, Godfraind J (1987) Competitive and stereoselective antagonistic effect of cicletanine in guinea-pig isolated ileum. Eur J Pharmacol 136: 235–240

231. Schölkens B (1978) Antihypertensive effect of prostacyclin (PGI_2) in experimental hypertension and its influence on plasma renin activity in rats. Prostagland Med 1: 359–372

232. Schölkens B, Steinbach R, Ganten D (1979) Blood pressure effects of endogenous brain angiotensin in rats are increased by inhibition of prostaglandin biosynthesis. Clin Sci 57: 271s–274s

233. Schölkens B, Gehring D, Schlotte V, Weithmann U (1982) Evening primose oil, a dietary prostaglandin precursor, diminishes vascular reactivity to renin and angiotensin II in rats. Prostagland Leukotr Med 8: 273–285

234. Schölkens B (1985) Prostaglandine. In: Ganten D, Ritz E (Hrsg) Lehrbuch der Hypertonie. Schattauer, Stuttgart New York, S 215–230

235. Schrör K (1984) Prostaglandine und verwandte Verbindungen. Bildung, Funktion und pharmakologische Beeinflussung. Thieme, Stuttgart New York

236. Seid JM, Jones PBB, Russell RGG (1983) The presence in normal plasma serum and platelets of factors that stimulate the production of prostacyclin (PGI_2) by cultured endothelial cells. Clin Sci 64: 387–394

237. Sell LL, Cullen ML, Lerner GR, Whittlesely GC, Shanly CJ, Klein MD (1987) Hypertension during extracorporeal membrane oxygenation: Cause, effect, and management. Surgery 102: 724–730

238. Sharpe GL, Larsson KS, Thalme B (1975) Studies on the closure of the ductus arteriosus. XII. In utero effect of indomethacin and sodium salicylate in rats and rabbits. Prostaglandins 9: 585–596

239. Shebuski RJ, Aiken JW (1980) Angiotensin II stimulation of renal prostaglandin synthesis elevates circulating prostacyclin in the dog. J Cardiovasc Pharmacol 2: 667–677

240. Siegl AM, Smith JB, Silver MJ, Nicolaou KC, Ahern D (1979) Selective binding site for ^{3}H-prostacyclin on platelets. J Clin Invest 63: 215–220
241. Silberbauer K, Stanek B, Templ H (1982) Acute hypotensive effect of captopril in man modified by prostaglandin synthesis inhibition. Br J Clin Pharmacol 14: 87S–93S
242. Simpson PJ, Lucchesi BR (1987) Myocardial ischemia: The potential therapeutic role of prostacyclin and its analogues. In: Gryglewski RJ, Stock G (eds) Prostacyclin and its stable analogue iloprost. Springer, Berlin Heidelberg New York Tokyo, pp 179–194
243. Singer P, Wirth M, Gödeke W, Heine H (1985) Blood pressure lowering effect of eicosapentaenoic acid – rich diet in normotensive, hypertensive and hyperlipidemic subjects. Experienta 41: 462–464
244. Sinzinger H, Fitscha P (1987) Prostaglandintherapie bei arteriellen Durchblutungsstörungen. Hämostaseologie 7: 120–127
245. Skidgel RA, Printz MP (1987) PGI_2 production in rat blood vessels: diminished prostacyclin formation in veins compared to arteries. Prostaglandins 16: 1–16
246. Skuballa W, Radüchel B, Vorbrüggen H (1987) Chemistry of stable prostacyclin analogues: Synthesis of iloprost. In Gryglewski RJ, Stock G (eds) Prostacyclin and its stable analogue iloprost. Springer, Berlin Heidelberg New York Tokyo, pp 17–24
247. Smith JB, Ogletree ML, Lefer AM (1978) Antibodies which antagonise the effects of prostacyclin. Nature 274: 64–65
248. Spokas EG, Quilley J, McGiff JC (1983) Prostaglandins in hypertension. In: Genest J, Kuchel O, Hamet P, Cantin M (eds) Hypertension physiopathology and treatment, 2nd edn. McGraw-Hill, New York St. Louis San Francisco, pp 373–390
249. Srivastava KC (1986) Effects of dipyridamole, nifedipine, verapamil, hydralazine and propranolol on the formation of prostacyclin and thromboxane in a coupled system of platelets and aorta. Prostagland Leuk Med 23: 31–36
250. Starling MB, Elbott RB (1974) The effects of prostaglandins, prostaglandin inhibitors, and oxygen on the closure of the ductus arteriosus, pulmonary arteries and umbilical vessels in vitro. Prostaglandins 8: 187–203
251. Stone KJ, Hart M (1976) Inhibition of renal PGE_2-9-ketoreductase by diuretics. Prostaglandins 12: 197–207
252. Sullivan JM, Patrick DR (1981) Release of prostaglandin I_2-like activity from the rat aorta: Effect of captopril, furosemide, and sodium. Prostaglandins 22: 575–585
253. Sun FF, Chapman JP, McGuire JC (1977) Metabolism of prostaglandin endoperoxide in animal tissues. Prostaglandins 14: 1055–1075
254. Sindar S (1987) Prostacyclin in (extracted) plasma of essential hypertensives Acta Cardiol 42: 135–139
255. Swartz SL, Williams GH, Hollenberg NK, Crantz FR, Levine L, Morre TJ, Dluhy RG (1980) Increase in prostaglandins during converting enzyme inhibition. Clin Sci 59: 133s–135s
256. Szczeklik A, Skawinski S, Gluszko P, Nizankowski R, Szczeklik J, Gryglewski RJ (1979) Successful therapy of advanced arteriosclerosis obliterans with prostacyclin. Lancet I: 1111–1115

257. Tan SY, Sweet P, Mulrow PJ (1978) Impaired renal production of prostaglandin E_2: A newly identified lesion in human essential hypertension. Prostaglandins 15: 139–558

258. Tarrade T, Guinot P (1988) Efficacy and tolerance of cicletanine, a new antihypertensive agent: Overview of 1226 treated patients. Drug Exp Clin Res 14: 205–214

259. Terashita Z, Fukui H, Nishikawa K, Hirata M, Kikuchi S (1982) Effects of arachidonic acid and bradykinin on the coronary flow, release of PGI_2 and cardiac functions in the perfused guinea-pig heart. Jap J Pharmacol 32: 351–358

260. Terragno NA, Terragno A, McGiff JC (1977) Contribution of prostaglandins to the renal circulation in conscious, anaesthetized and laparatomized dogs. Circ Res 40: 590–595

261. Terragno NA, McGiff JC, Snugel M, Terragno A (1978) Patterns of prostaglandin production in the bovine fetal and maternal vasculature. Prostaglandins 16: 843–855

262. Ts'ao C (1970) Tissue-specific induction of platelet aggregation in vitro. Am J Pathol 61: 75–78

263. Tschopp TB, Baumgartner HR (1982) Prostacyclin (PGI_2) aus Gefäßmuskelzellen hemmt Plättchenadhäsion und -aggregation auf dem Subendothel von Arterien. In: van de Loo J, Asbeck F (eds) Hämostase, Thrombophilie und Arteriosklerose. Schattauer, Stuttgart, S 489–492

264. Udermann HD, Jackson EK, Puett D, Workman RJ (1984) Thromboxane synthetase inhibitor UK38,485 lowers blood pressure in the adult spontaneously hypertensive rat. J Cardiovasc Pharmacol 6: 969–972

265. Uehara Y, Ishii M, Ikeda T, Atarashi K, Takeda T, Murao S (1983) Plasma levels of 6-keto-prostaglandin $F_{1\alpha}$ in normotensive subjects and patients with essential hypertension. Prostagland Leukotr Med 10: 455–464

266. Uehara Y, Tobian L, Iwai J, Ishii M, Sugimoto T (1987) Alterations of vascular prostacyclin and thromboxane A_2 in Dahl genetical strain suspectible to salt-induced hypertension. Prostaglandins 33: 727–739

267. Valone FH, Johnson B (1987) Modulation of platelet-activating-factor-induced calcium influx and intracellular calcium release by phorbol esters. Biochem J 247: 669–674

268. Vandongen R, O'Dwyer J, Barden A (1983) Release of prostaglandins during reversal of one-kidney, but not two-kidney, one-clip hypertension in the rat. J Hypertens 1: 177–182

269. Vandongen R, McGowan H, Anderson H, Barden A (1985) Renal prostanoids after unclipping the denervated one-kidney, one-clip hypertensive rat. Am J Physiol 249: F542–F545

270. Vane JR, McGiff JC (1975) Possible contributions of endogenous prostaglandins to the control of blood pressure. Circ Res Suppl I, 36 and 37: I-68–I-75

271. Vargaftig BB, Dao Hai N (1972) Selective inhibition by mepacrine of the release of "rabbit aorta contracting substance" evoked by the administration of bradykinin. J Pharm Pharmacol 24: 159–161

272. Verberckmoes R, van Damme B, Clement J, Amery A, Michielsen P (1976) Bartter's syndrome with hyperplasia of renomedullary cells: Successful treatment with indomethacin. Kidney Int 9: 302–307

273. Vierhapper H, Waldhäusl W, Nowotny P (1981) Effect of indomethacin upon angiotensin-induced changes in blood pressure and plasma aldosterone in normal man. Eur J Clin Invest 11: 85–89

274. Vinci JM, Horowitz D, Zusmann RM, Pisano JJ, Catt KJ, Keiser HR (1979) The effect of converting enzyme inhibition with SQ 20881 on plasma and urinary kinins, prostaglandin E and angiotensin II in hypertensive man. Hypertension 1: 416–426

275. Vio CP, Churchill L, Terragno A, McGiff JC, Terragno NA (1982) Arachidonic acid stimulates renal kallikrein release in isolated rat kidney. Clin Sci 63: 235s–237s

276. Vlasses PH, Ferguson RK, Smith JB, Rotmensch HH, Swanson BN (1983) Urinary excretion of prostacyclin and thromboxane A_2 metabolites after angiotensin converting enzyme inhibition in hypertensive patients. Prostagland Leukotr Med 11: 143–150

277. Wallenburg HC, Makovitz W, Dekker GA, Rotmans P (1986) Low dose aspirin prevents pregnancy induced hypertension and pre-eclampsia in angiotensin sensitive primigravida. Lancet I: 1–3

278. Walsh WS (1985) Pre-eclampsia: An imbalance in placental prostacyclin and thromboxane production. Am J Obstet Gynecol 152: 335–340

279. Watkins J, Abbott EC, Hensby CN, Webster J (1980) Attenuation of hypotensive effect of propranolol and thiazide diuretics by indomethacin. Brit Med J 281: 702–707

280. Weber PC, Larrson C, Änggard E, Hamberg M, Corey EJ, Nicolaou KC, Samuelsson (1976) Stimulation of renin release from rabbit renal cortex by arachidonic acid and prostaglandin endoperoxides. Circ Res 39: 868–874

281. Weber PC, Scherer B, Held E, Siess W, Stoffel H (1979) Urinary prostaglandins and kallikrein in essential hypertension Clin Sci 57: 259s–261s

282. Weber PC, Siess W, Scherer B (1979) Vaskuläre, thrombozytäre und renale Prostaglandine. Biochemie, Funktion, klinische Aspekte. Klin Wochenschr 57: 425–444

283. Weber PC, Siess W, Scherer B, Held E, Witzgall H, Lorenz R (1982) Arachidonic acid metabolites, hypertension and arteriosclerosis. Klin Wochenschr 60:479–488

284. Webster J, Dollery CT, Hensby CN, Friedman LA (1980) Antihypertensive action of bendroflumethiazide: Increased prostacyclin production? Clin Pharmacol Ther 28: 751–758

285. Weeks JR, Compton LD (1979) The cardiovascular pharmacology of prostacyclin (PGI_2) in the rat. Prostaglandins 17: 501–513

286. Weithmann KU (1980) The influence of pentoxifylline on interaction between blood vessel wall and platelets. IRCS Med Sci 8: 293–294

287. Weksler BB, Knapp JM, Jaffe EA (1977) Prostacyclin (PGI_2) synthesized by cultured endothelial cells modulates polymorphonuclear leukocyte function. Blood 50 (Suppl 1): 287

288. Weksler BB, Ley CW, Jaffe EA (1978) Stimulation of endothelial cell prostacyclin production by thrombin, trypsin, and ionophore-A-23187. J Clin Invest 63: 923–930

289. Weksler BB (1982) Prostacyclin. In: Spact TH (ed) Progress in hemostasis and thrombosis, Vol 6. Grune & Stratton, New York, pp 113–138

290. Wennmalm Ä (1978) Influence of indomethacin on the systemic and pulmonary vascular resistance in man. Clin Sci Mol Med 54: 141–145

291. Wennmalm Ä, Brundin T (1978) Prostaglandin-mediated inhibition of noradrenaline release. IV. Prostaglandin synthesis is stimulated by myocardial adrenoceptors differing from the α- and β-type. Acta Physiol Scand 102: 374–381

292. Whittle BJR, Higgs GA, Eakins KE, Moncada S, Vane JR (1980) Selective inhibition of prostaglandin production in inflammatory exudates and gastric mucosa. Nature 184: 271–273

293. Whorton AR, Misono K, Hollifield J, Frölich JC, Inagami T, Oates JA (1977) Prostaglandins and renin release: I. Stimulation of renin release from rabbit renal cortical slices by PGI_2. Prostaglandins 14: 1095–1104

294. Whorton AR, Young SU, Data JL, Barchowsky A, Kent RS (1982) Mechanism of bradykinin-stimulated prostacyclin synthesis in porcine aortic endothelial cells. Biochim Biophys Acta 712: 79–87

295. Windeck R, Brodde O-E (1988) Stimulation des Renin-Aldosteron-Systems durch Prostacyclininfusion bei hyporeninämischen Hypoaldosteronismus. Med Klin 83: 289–291

296. Wing LMH, Bune AJC, Chalmers JP, Graham JR, West MJ (1981) The effects of indomethacin treated hypertensive patients. Clin Exp Pharmacol Physiol 8: 537–541

297. Witzgall H, Hirsch F, Scherer B, Weber PC (1982) Acute haemodynamic and hormonal effects of captopril are diminished by indomethacin. Clin Sci 62: 611–615

298. Wlodawer P, Hammarström S (1979) Some properties of prostacyclin synthetase from pig aorta. Biochim Biophys Acta 97: 33–36

299. Wong PYK, Malik KU, Desiderio DM, McGiff JC, Sun FF (1980) Hepatic metabolism of prostacyclin (PGI_2) in the rabbit: formation of a potent novel inhibitor of platelet aggregation. Biochem Biophys Res Commun 93: 486–494

300. Ylitalo P, Pitkäjärvi T, Metsä-Ketelä T, Vapaatalo H (1978) The effect of inhibition of prostaglandin synthesis on plasma renin activity and blood pressure in essential hypertension. Prostagland Med 1: 479–488

301. Ylitalo P, Kaukinen S, Nurmi A-E, Seppälä E, Pessi T, Vapaatalo H (1985) Effects of a prostacyclin analog iloprost on kidney function, renin-angiotensin and kallikrein-kinin systems, prostanoids and catecholamines in man. Prostaglandins 29: 1063–1071

302. Zavoico GB, Feinstein MB (1984) Cytoplasmatic calcium in platelets is controlled by cyclic AMP: Antagonism between stimulators and inhibitors of adenylate cyclase. Biochim Biophys Res Comm 120: 579–585

303. Zusman RM (1983) Regulation of prostaglandin biosynthesis in cultured renal medullary interstitial cells. In: Dunn MJ, Patrono C, Cinotti GA (eds) Prosta-

glandins and the kidneys. Biochemistry, physiology, pharmacology, and clinical applications. Plenum, New York London, pp 17–25

304. Zusman RM (1984) Renin- and non-renin-mediated antihypertensive actions of converting enzyme inhibitors. Kidney Int 25: 969–983

Index

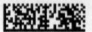